SOUNDINGS

SOUNDINGS
FROM BMJ COLUMNISTS

Articles from the *British Medical Journal*
Published by the BMJ Publishing Group
Tavistock Square, London WC1H 9JR

First published 1992

British Library Cataloguing-in-
Publication Data.
A catalogue record for this book is
available from the British Library.

ISBN 0-7279-0776 X

Printed and bound in Great Britain by
Latimer Trend & Company Ltd., Plymouth

Contents

COLIN DOUGLAS, *doctor and novelist, Edinburgh*

JAMES OWEN DRIFE, *professor of obstetrics and gynaecology, University of Leeds*

GEORGE DUNEA, *attending physician, Cook County Hospital, Chicago*

TONY SMITH, *associate editor, BMJ*

DAVID WIDGERY, *general practitioner, London*

Introduction

I once heard a pub philosopher in Worcester remark, sagely (they are always sage—it's in the job description), "Christmas has to be paid for; that can't be swept under the carpet." At the time I put this homespun version of "There's no such thing as a free lunch" down to west midlands dourness rather than recognition of an essential fact of life, but it turns out like most truisms to be true—and this book is a case in point.

As a senior member of the *BMJ*'s editorial staff (and I use senior as in senior citizen—viz aged—rather than in today's more common usage of Seriously Important) I have among my editorial tasks to edit the page called "Soundings," in which regular contributors expound wittily and/or passionately on life, the universe, and everything pertaining to medical practice and the world at large. I do not spread it around, but this job is a piece of cake: the contributors all write like angels, they deliver their pieces on time, are all charming to deal with and, apart from a propensity to involve the *BMJ* in expensive and acrimonious libel suits, entirely without fault.

But the downside has emerged, and in spades. From a year's worth of articles I now have to select a minority for this anthology.

I decided to take into account something that has struck me over the years when dealing with doctors at what you might call the business end of the trade rather than the literary one. I mean GPs and hospital consultants, when I have had to consult them. They may be glacially efficient or cosily caring, do nameless things to your person or simply tell you to take more exercise/rest/tonic with the gin, but sooner or later they come round to the dreaded question:

"What do you do for a living?"

"I work on the *BMJ*."

At this point the medical person will snort, smirk, blush, or grin apologetically. But they all say the same thing: "Oh, I never read that—I don't understand it."

Presumably they have been saying the same thing to ED, *BMJ* because a couple of years ago he resolved to make the last six pages of the journal the medical equivalent of a colour supplement—the bit you relax with after the hard core science. Being an upmarket publication we don't have royal college love-nest scandals or the memoirs of Nazi doctors, we have comment, reviews and, best of all (I would say that, wouldn't I?) "Soundings."

This collection of "Soundings" pieces, therefore, is for all those doctors who don't understand the *BMJ*, for those who do, and for the families, friends, and perhaps patients of both kinds. I don't think you will find many recurring themes among the writers: they are a mixed bunch and their subjects range from chilblains to Third World debt, from fire alarms to self prescribing by chimpanzees. There does come up from many of the pages, though, a whiff of melancholy at the state of the National Health Service and what is being done to it; in David Widgery's polemics and Colin Douglas's vignettes you feel the pain of those working in a profession which, if not in crisis, is certainly in a terrible state of chassis. The pressure of market forces on health services also comes under George Dunea's ironic scrutiny in Chicago. You will find different aspects of doctors as human beings explored, forcefully by Trisha Greenhalgh and with high comedy by Julie Welch. James Owen Drife will bring you out alternately in belly-laughs and goose-pimples, while Tony Smith and Bernard Dixon will illuminate, inform, and broaden your mind.

But why try to classify them? they can speak for themselves. I have therefore grouped the articles under author, alphabetically—except that in a fit of political incorrectness I have put the ladies first. Enjoy.

RUTH HOLLAND
BMJ

Trisha Greenhalgh

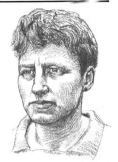

EAVESDROPPING

There is a redundant chair in the back reception area, out of
sight of the waiting room but within earshot. The other day I
was sitting there reading the post when a woman came in to ask for
an urgent appointment.

"Dr Greenhalgh in 10 minutes?" offered the receptionist.

"Er, no. Anyone but Dr Greenhalgh, please."

"Hmm. Take a seat, then, and be prepared to wait."

The patient seated herself inches from my hidden ears. "After
what she said about my little boy . . . absolute indictment . . .
reflects on the whole family . . . and he's a lovely lad, the brightest
of the three in fact."

(*Good grief, what did I say?*)

An old lady came to my rescue. "Well, she's always been very
nice to me. She let me have an *x* ray after Dr T said I didn't need
one. . . ."

(*Shaky grounds for accolade, but you didn't come back for four
months.*)

"All over his notes she wrote it, and on the outside."

". . . and she gave me a lift home in her car once."

"They get paid for that."

(*No, we don't.*)

"She's only got an old Fiat. I thought they all had posh cars."

(*Well, there you are.*)

"She's married to one of the specialists at the hospital. . . ."

(*No, I'm not.*)

"I saw her in Tesco's once. It's amazing what they buy."

(*Eggs, pasta, shampoo. What's amazing about that?*)

"She only works three mornings a week."

(*I only get paid for three mornings a week.*)

". . . I came over queer the other night and I didn't know how to get hold of a doctor. . . ."

(*Try reading the practice leaflet.*)

". . . of course, her name isn't in the phone book. . . ."

(*Yes it is, but I'm glad you can't spell it.*)

". . . in the end I had a hot lemon and it all passed over."

(*Hah!*)

"She doesn't give you anything, anyway. You can be waiting here two hours sometimes and she'll still say you don't need anything. . . ."

(*Keep talking.*)

". . . you ask the chemist for something and the chemist will tell you to see the doctor, and then she'll tell you to go back to the chemist. . . ."

(*I say, "If you really feel the need to take something, you could ask the chemist."*)

"I had a boil on me private, and she said just leave it alone. . . ."

(*And you didn't, did you?*)

". . . you don't like going to them with things down there. You don't know who they'll tell."

(*Probably not the whole waiting room.*)

Time to start surgery. On my way out I checked some notes. Goodness, she was right. In my handwriting, in large black letters, reproduced on the outer jacket, were the deathless words ASTHMATIC CHILD.

HEARTSINK AND ROSES

His 20 minutes were up, but he did not budge. He was a small man. Arthritis had medicalised him to the point where he was at ease in my surgery and the local teaching hospital, but never elsewhere. He had what I call a personality disorder; my mother would call it a chip on the shoulder. Most of his friends, including a doting girlfriend, were fictional. His visits to me for trivial complaints had gradually become unacceptably frequent. He had firmly refused psychiatric referral, and my attempts at confrontational psychotherapy had been a disaster. We now had a truce. He made a double appointment once a month and presented a discourse on his current symptoms, while I doodled on my blotter and planned what to give the kids for tea. It went down in the notes as "gen chat." On a good day I thought of it as counselling; on a bad day, timewasting.

He was not allowed to go over time. I cleared my throat and repeated my recommendation to "take more rest." He leant forward so that his knee was touching mine and said, "My idea of a good rest, my dear, is lying between silk sheets and making love to a sweet young lady such as yourself." Interpreting my numb silence as encouragement, he continued, "I'm sure a gorgeous girl like you isn't short of offers . . . you probably never thought of me as good in bed. . . ." His hand closed over mine.

I am not as swarthy as the sketch here suggests, but I am no bit of fluff. In previous encounters with aspiring rapists I have outrun one, knocked a second unconscious, and dealt a sizable scrotal haematoma to the third. The local flasher had once hurriedly rezipped himself after I scorned the size of his organ. I was nearly twice the size of my current aggressor, 10 years his senior, and trained in martial arts. In any case, I was being propositioned, not attacked. Yet in 30 seconds this epitome of inadequacy had reduced me to a crimson, trembling wreck. With ill feigned dignity I stalked out of the room and locked myself in the ladies, leaving the receptionist to evict the patient.

Sexual harassment is a power game, with one party playing on the other's real or perceived role of victim. Responding with verbal or physical aggression explodes the game by rejecting the victim role. But such behaviour is constrained by professional obligations. The consultation, too, is a power game. With heartsink patients, it becomes an almighty battle. Passive, dependent patients push us into the parent role to realise their own fantasy role of favoured child. This is often the only way to manage them. But the illusion of control over a heartsink patient (as over a recalcitrant child) depends heavily on keeping one's cool.

My pathetic, crippled patient had succeeded where his more credible predecessors had failed. He had forced me to choose between a behaviour compatible with my professional role and one which responded effectively to his sexual impropriety. In choosing the first, I had unwittingly become his victim.

A GAUNTLET FOR SENIOR HOUSE OFFICERS

M y first call as a trainee general practitioner was to a 23 year old man with pyrexia of unknown origin. Two days earlier he had been discharged from hospital with a diagnosis of "viral illness with social problems and functional overlay." I was sent to placate the family and investigate the hidden agenda. I found the patient semiconscious, shocked, and delirious. On readmission he was found to have disseminated tuberculosis.

He was lucky. The medical senior house officer had listened to me. A friend of mine, an experienced general practitioner, recently visited a 70 year old diabetic man with severe breathlessness. He was pyrexial and confused, and one lung field was obscured by what was probably a large pleural effusion. The patient lived on the third floor of a council block with an invalid wife and psychotic daughter, neither of whom could get to the phone or make a cup of tea.

My friend telephoned the local teaching hospital to request a medical admission. It was the first week in August. The admitting senior house officer told her to administer a diuretic and call back in the morning. My friend stated that she did not think the problem was heart failure. The senior house officer suggested she try an antibiotic. My friend (who has more postgraduate qualifications than this young man is ever likely to obtain) stated that in her opinion the patient needed further investigation, close observation, and nursing care. The senior house officer thought these services could be provided by the general practitioner herself and the district nurses, but promised to discuss the problem with his registrar. He did not ring back.

My friend arranged the man's admission through channels open only to that fortunate minority of general practitioners who know the consultant socially. The story has become a favourite dinner party anecdote. Perhaps some other member of that cocky breed of on-take senior house officers who have been qualified a year and a day might like to bolster his or her curriculum vitae by conducting a controlled trial of general practitioner admission requests. The result might read as follows:

"One hundred consecutive requests for medical admission by general practitioners were assessed by a senior house officer. On the basis of the telephone information provided by the general practitioner the request was classified as appropriate or inappropriate. All patients were then seen in casualty and assessed by an experienced clinician. It was found that 15% of the requests for admission had been appropriate, and that all of these had been correctly identified over the telephone by the senior house officer. Of the remaining requests 25% were caused primarily by clinical incompetence on the part of the general practitioner, 30% by laziness, and 20% by an underhand attempt to jump the queue for an outpatient appointment. It was concluded that the patronising of general practitioners by the most junior ranks of hospital doctor is entirely justified, and that the assessment over the telephone of apparently very sick patients by these junior doctors is an accurate and reliable method of clinical triage."

CASES FOR FINALS

In early spring, when the evenings lengthen and the buds begin to open, the thoughts of the young registrar turn to finding suitable cases for the final MB examination. The cases will not actually be needed until midsummer, and therein lies a tale.

A few years ago it was my lot to organise the short cases. I waited with my clipboard for the arrival by minicab of what promised to be a walking gallery of exotic physical signs. The first patient suffered from myelofibrosis. I showed her to her cubicle and asked if I might examine her to confirm what was on the card. "Oh, you won't need to do that, dear, it hasn't rubbed off yet," she said. Her abdomen bore the unmistakable signs of a recent teaching session with the junior students. An enlarged liver and spleen, complete with notch, were delineated in thick black ink. I phoned round in search of some ethyl alcohol and resited her in the examiners' tea room.

Patient two was a military type with a dark blue blazer who introduced himself as the RVO. He began to instil his own mydriatics. Cracking the acronym, I reached for my ophthalmoscope. His fundi were normal. The boss breezed in, confirmed that my gentleman now had a retinal vein occlusion (resolved), and breezed out. Patient three, a boy with Down's syndrome and Fallot's tetralogy, arrived with a rather gormless nanny and started to play with the instruments. Every time I touched him with my stethoscope he chanted "ninety-nine, ninety-nine, ninety-nine" at the top of his voice until I removed it again. I didn't try asking him to squat.

The two psychiatric cases arrived together. Careful questioning revealed a striking absence of first rank symptoms, mood disturbance, or personality disorder in either of them. So much for modern neuroleptics. The woman with polycystic kidneys rang in sick; the cab driver had been unable to find the man with Marfan's syndrome; and the girl with mitral valve prolapse was diverted to casualty with a panic attack.

It was 10 minutes to curtain up and so far the only hard physical sign I had seen all morning was the external examiner's rhinophyma. That was clearly out of bounds, as was the home professor's mental state, which in the presence of attractive female students was reputed to border on the psychopathic. I knew the nurse was breastfeeding, but appearing as a case of galactorrhoea was clearly beyond the call of duty. Ditto for the cleaning lady's varicose veins.

The senior registrar was an old hand at this game. "Happens every year," he murmured. Eight minutes later the cubicles were almost all occupied. The RVO was bearing his smoker's chest; the hyperactive Down's child had become a psychiatric/social case; the lady with myelofibrosis reappeared complete with an allergic reaction to the cleaning fluid, and the recuperated schizophrenic patient sat contemplating his newly discovered carotid bruit. "We just need one more case," said the senior registrar. As he looked at me his eyes lit up. "Just put your chin up and swallow. . . . Yes!

Take a seat behind that curtain, madam. We'll scan your thyroid after the show."

WARD OF SHAME

My earliest memory is of a picnic in a park near Alder Hey Hospital in Liverpool, and then days of darkness. Eyes bandaged, I followed the hospital routine by sound and smell. I remember a sweet and sour mixture of carbolic, bitter medicine, comfort food, scoldings, lullabies, and gentle unbuttoning hands. The shrill bell that banished one's parents was a nuisance, but a forlorn toddler, sprouting pigtails from bandaged head, could count on being swept up in a starchy embrace by many a passing nurse. It was a ward of darkness but not of malice, and I was left with no permanent scars.

My next five admissions were all orthopaedic. I cannot do flicflacs, cycle round corners, or ice skate, but I have collected some good scars trying. In orthopaedic wards the macho lie mending, the daredevil exchange stories of their collision courses, and pretty nurses suffer endless sexual harassment. They are wards of revelry, where most of the injuries are self inflicted but no one feels guilty or ashamed.

Today, I am on the gynaecology ward. I have hyperemesis gravidarum. I lie here wired up to my drip and feel guilty. I am neglecting work, home, family, and friends. Three of the other patients have had miscarriages—one from cycling to work, one through sexual intercourse, and one after a previous termination of pregnancy. Another woman's hysterectomy scar burst open when she was pegging the washing out. The woman who had an intrauterine death is guilty twice over—for giving birth to a dead child and for not having the courage to look at it before they took it away. The woman having injections for infertility is getting all the right treatment but her body is not responding.

The whole ward is enveloped in a pervasive sense of shame. We are bad mothers; we are women gone bad.

The womb was once thought of as the centre of a woman's

7

consciousness. The feminist in me resents a definition of herself in terms solely of wife, mother, and lover. The rationalist in me explains my illness as a quirk of physiology, no more my fault than a sprained ankle. Then whence this melancholy?

In recent weeks I have gained much insight from a friend whose habit of explaining life's ups and downs in terms of the phases of the moon used to irritate me. I had never taken seriously her theory that "womb-consciousness" is a whole dimension of spirituality unique to the female sex: in health the source of some mystical womanly strength, and in sickness the soul's deepest torment. Without realising it, I had dismissed the tears of my premenstrual, infertile, and perimenopausal patients as expressions of a general weakness of character. I had always argued that well man clinics were more logical on clinical grounds than well woman clinics.

This illness has taught me a new lesson. Gynaecological health is inseparable from psychic health. The soul hurts and bleeds with the womb. Management of a gynaecological problem is incomplete without management of the psychic distress that inevitably accompanies it. The shame must be recognised and treated as well as the pain.

AUTIE'S TRIAL

A family friend, whom I have always called Auntie, rings up regularly to inform me of developments in her medical problems. Last month there was some exciting news. Auntie had Blood Pressure and had been asked to help with a large trial comparing one new drug with another. Did I approve? I thought it was a splendid idea. So, apparently, did her other unpaid medical advisers—a chiropodist and a retired eye surgeon. Auntie signed up.

Blood pressure is a fickle affliction. Next day there was a call to say she didn't have it any more and unless it came back she was out of the game. But a fortnight later Auntie stood triumphantly on my doorstep bearing a list of blood pressure readings on the back of a bus ticket and a bar coded white box. She thought she had better take the first tablet in my front room, just in case. And she had been given a questionnaire which I was to help her fill in. I put the kettle on.

The questionnaire weighed about half a pound. The patient was optimistically informed that it would take 30 minutes to complete 27 pages of questions on his or her health, lifestyle, and attitudes. The envelope was marked "Confidential: your answers on this form will not be seen by your general practitioner." This sentence caused Auntie visible distress. She had expected that her responses would be carefully perused by her trusted family doctor. She awarded him nine out of ten for the question "How useful is he/she in giving advice about your health?" (as "family and friends" I got three out of ten). To the question "Has your general practitioner discussed any of the following with you in the last three months . . .?" she ticked all the boxes: diet, smoking, alcohol, stress. I was surprised, since Auntie neither smokes nor drinks. She gave me a dark look. "If he thought it was necessary he would discuss it."

Over supper, Auntie confided that she would probably live to a ripe old age because she looked after herself, ate the right sort of margarine and attended a keep fit class, and because her mother had lived to 88. Yet on the Health Knowledge section ("The following things influence my health. . .") Auntie answered "don't know" to every question. She did not want to say yes in case it was the wrong answer.

She did, however, lay claim to some stressful life events. The gas bill apparently counted as a "severe financial tragedy." Then there was the "death of a close relative or friend." A lady at church had passed away (aged 96) a few months back, and judging from the visual analogue scale, Auntie had found this overwhelmingly distressing. It would, she said, have been disrespectful to the dead to have put her cross anywhere else.

Auntie thinks that the aim of the faceless statisticians who analyse her answers is to check up on her general practitioner. I know better. Their aim is to publish a paper drawing erudite conclusions about the influence of a host of existential and psychometric variables on the response to treatment of essential hypertension, based entirely on the answers to one lengthy and indigestible questionnaire. I wish them luck.

Julie Welch

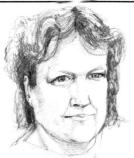

DOCTORS' DISCRETION

"Isn't it interesting," I commented recently to a friend, "how journalists and doctors are completely different personality types?"

"What makes you think," snapped my friend, "that doctors have any personality at all?" He is married to a GP who had been called out at night three Saturdays on the trot and may have been a little miffed at the lack of dinner on the table.

However, I think I'm right. For instance, I went to 11 parties over Christmas and the New Year and they all had one thing in common. It was never the GPs who stayed up till 4.30 in the morning singing "Nessun dorma." The doctors weren't the ones who fell off their seats at the formal dinner nor did they settle disputes over who ought to be picked at centre forward for Scotland by punching the daylights out of each other. I say thank God for the medical profession. Journalists, book people, and theatricals might be a tad livelier when it comes to having a turn at the karaoke machine, but you can always rely on doctors to keep their clothes on and refrain from ruining anyone else's by pouring wine over them in a fit of sexual jealousy.

If I remember correctly from "Introduction to Psychology" during my first year at university, the term for such doctors is stable introvert. This is not to say that at home they don't have a den in which they dress up as Elvis and mime to his greatest hits, but out there in the social whirl they make the ideal guests— quietly spoken, moderate in their habits, clearing up the debris made by other people. If journalists and other creative types are eternal children then doctors are eternal parents.

Journalists are naive and pompous enough to believe that what they think is important or at least entertaining, whereas the doctors I meet seem increasingly to feel disillusioned and ineffective. Both groups are, however, alike in one thing. In the course of their jobs they have to interview people. In the doctor's case this is to diagnose, and in the journalist's case to expose.

In each instance there is an interaction between two people, and both doctor and journalist must observe, ask personal questions, and make notes. Here the similarity ends, particularly if the journalist works for a tabloid newspaper. The doctor keeps the patient's answers to herself and, using her observations, attempts to alleviate the problem. The hack, on the other hand, promptly shares the details of the transaction with a million readers and leaves the interviewee high and dry to cope with whatever scandal, censure, or ridicule that may result. A doctor never reinvents or embroiders a patient's symptoms to make them sound more exciting, whereas if a hack thinks that what you have told him doesn't square with the story he wants to write he will just make it up.

Journalists are the world's most dedicated gossips. They are flamboyantly indiscreet about passing on what they've seen or heard and would shop their own grandmothers if it made good copy. Doctors, on the other hand, are by nature and training inclined to keep everyone's secrets safe. That is why they are perfect for parties. Whatever gross misbehaviour takes place before their eyes, they will never tell a soul.

NEXT, PLEASE

I have a boil on my chin—no, honestly, this is not an appeal for sympathy—which may necessitate a visit to the doctor. I say "may" because nowadays you feel duty bound to work out whether such a visit is worthy of his/her time.

The days are gone when you woke in the morning feeling as if someone were using a road drill on your head, and staggered down to the surgery to demand your prescription. This usually got you a bottle of something called The Linctus, which was the colour of traffic lights and tasted of crushed barley sugar held together by wallpaper paste. It was so foul you ended up pouring it down the sink, and your head got better by itself.

Nowadays you think twice about visiting the surgery. The responsibility is terrifying. Can the National Health afford to dispense this medicine to me? Hasn't the doctor got enough on her plate without listening to me wittering on about my boil/stiff neck/tendency to weep uncontrollably upon hearing ancient Beatles hits? Why don't I just stay at home and take paracetamol?

The decision tends to be influenced by which doctors are on duty at our six quack practice. Dr A, for instance, is lovely. Despite being married with her own young family, she actually volunteers to pay house calls at weekends, which makes you feel so guilty you'd drop dead rather than drag her out. The only drawback about Dr A is, of course, her very desirability. Everyone else wants to see her too. She is booked up almost as far ahead as *Cats* and *Aspects of Love*. Fine if you've got something that will wait but if you're suffering from chest pains it is probably best to look elsewhere.

The receptionist may suggest booking you in with Dr B. Visiting him is reassuringly predictable. You go in and tell him your symptoms, he scratches his head and says, "I wonder what that can be." For this reason it's best to offer him little hints or pointers before you start, like, "I'm eight months pregnant." I know that doctors are attempting to take themselves off their pedestals, but sometimes I think he may be going a little too far.

There is no danger of iatrogenic illness with Dr B. Whatever is wrong with you, he will smile kindly and say, "There's nothing you can take for it, but come back in a week if you're no better." The main advantage of Dr B is availability. No one wants to see him, so you can get an appointment at short notice.

Sometimes I think back wistfully to the doctor I met on a chartered aeroplane in my days as a football reporter. He was employed by the first division club we had just watched lose by two goals in Europe. It was late at night, and the plane, crowded with players, officials, press, and a number of selected fans, began its descent into a fog-shrouded Luton Airport. I think we must have

13

been about ten feet off the ground when the engines roared and we headed rapidly upwards again. We circled. The second attempt at landing took place. That, too, was aborted at the last moment. Dumb and rigid with fear, we gripped the seat rests as the pilot took us round for the third time.

One of the fans could bear it no longer. "We're all going to die," he wailed. The stewardess hurried to his aid and with a concerned expression beckoned for the club doctor. He rushed up to the stricken passenger, examined him, and gestured to the stewardess to fetch a drink. She ran back with a glass of brandy and handed it to the doctor, who swallowed it in one gulp. I'd love to know what he prescribes for boils on the chin.

A HEALTHY PERSONALITY

I went to Aintree the other week for the Grand National. Racing people aren't like the rest of us. For a start, they don't watch much racing. It is possible to attend an entire meeting without moving away from the bar—inhaling tobacco fumes and ducking flying champagne corks. The thunder of hooves on turf is drowned out by the glug-glug-glug of people drinking and the crash of breaking glasses. This is punctuated by the occasional burst of aerobic exercise in which everyone rushes to the wall-mounted video screen, jumps up and down shouting, "Come on, you bugger!" for several minutes, then hurls crumpled betting slips to the floor. Real fitness fanatics may also get involved in a spot of impromptu brawling.

I was introduced to an elderly titled chap who had a treble Scotch in one hand and a cigar the size of a railway carriage in the other. "Only just come out of hospital," he confided. "Had a spot of surgery on me neck." This turned out to be some complicated and life-preserving operation on the carotid artery and it had taken place a mere two weeks previously. Still, he'd managed to demolish a bottle of whisky the previous night, hadn't got to bed till 4, felt a bit off colour now but mustn't grumble. It was a little hard to come up with an appropriate response; of all the comments which came to mind the politest was, "What a twit."

However, I had the great good fortune to meet up with my favourite travelling companion, a Glaswegian sportswriter employed by one of our national tabloid newspapers. He is known as Big 'Un, not out of any irony. He is six feet tall and jolly fat, with a red round beaming face. A 40 a day man, and almost always the last to leave the hostelry, he has pursued this lifestyle for at least 32 of his 50 years, getting bigger and redder by the year. His joyousness never flags.

After the final day's racing we couldn't find a taxi to take us back to Liverpool Lime Street, so we joined a crowd of several thousand on the platform of Aintree station, where we waited for half an hour, during which my friend joined energetically in a singsong with the locals. Our train to London Euston left Lime Street at 6.40, and the Aintree train deposited us at Liverpool Central at 6.35. We had five minutes. The whole trip was worth while just to see Big 'Un sprint the half mile between stations. I thought, This is it; this has got to be the end; he will keel over and die. But there he was, bobbing tantalisingly ahead of me like a great red marker buoy while I flagged with the nervous dyspepsia that had dogged me since the struggle to meet the first day's deadline. Okay, I may have had a hangover too.

Lime Street loomed in front of us. Big 'Un rounded the barrier, laid a restraining hand on the guard, and held open the carriage door for me. We got in. The train moved off, at which Big 'Un had a large cigar and a bottle of champagne to celebrate, and I went away and sat in a corner and tried not to throw up.

Why is my friend still alive and kicking? He loves his job, and he has a very happy marriage, though these may be effects rather than causes. I think he just has a healthy personality—an immense and continuing enjoyment of life, a curiosity and relish, a splendid combination of scepticism and romanticism, and a childlike ability to play. Mind you, I do think he could lose a couple of stone.

JULIE WELCH

A PROPER PROFESSION

My mother was very keen that I should be a doctor. Actually, she was very keen that my sister should be a doctor, but when Heather discovered that a career in medicine meant two thirds of a decade at university followed by a lifetime of 200 hour weeks, she said "Stuff that for a game of marbles" and went off to Paris to roar up and down the Champs Elysées in a Sunbeam Alpine with a rich, besotted comte. My mother's ambitions then devolved to me. At least one of her daughters should enjoy a proper professional title.

Unfortunately, a swift roll call of 150 years of Welches reveals pioneers of science, newspaper editors, botanists, pork butchers, army deserters, and sheep stealers but no doctors—evidence which may indicate that we are genetically disinclined for medicine. For a start, the women of our family are the kind who like to come into a room to the sound of ecstatic and prolonged applause, plus a 22 piece band. Jolly useful if you happen to be doing the closing number at the Royal Variety Performance but not, perhaps, a quality much appreciated by the clientele of a busy inner city general practice.

So, alas, I too disappointed her. The fact that, in our chosen spheres of education and the written word, both my big sister and I have spent our adult years working long and hard cuts no ice with my mother who, like the rest of the world, holds doctors in the kind of awe more properly reserved for great spiritual leaders and people who can hit six sixes off the West Indian pace attack. Even now, as I show her the dust jacket blurb for my first novel ("passionate, funny and utterly original"), I detect a tendency to sign and turn away and say, "Of course, I always hoped you would be a doctor."

I suspect it's an idea gleaned from the early days of commercial television, when *Emergency Ward 10* flickered across black and white screens in suburban homes up and down the country, forming the prototype for all medical soaps in perpetuity. I don't remember it in any detail; but for some reason I have inherited my mother's attitude. Whenever someone I meet socially says they are a doctor I take a step back and make a hasty mental replay of our conversation to see if I've said anything unsuitable. It's a bit like

16

talking to men of the cloth. I suppose it's because one thinks that, like the clergy, doctors are closer to the big issues of the human condition. When the Grim Reaper is about to drop by, you call in one if not the other.

This is probably why I found myself wondering the other day what doctors talk about when they are together. I imagined elevated conversations about, for instance, the ethical dilemmas caused by imposing a market discipline on the NHS. I got the chance to find out when my son's friend, the child of two White Coated Ones, came to stay for the weekend.

"Tell me," I said, "what kind of things do your parents discuss over the dinner table?"

"Urine samples," came the curt reply.

THROBBING IN THE DORM

During the sixties I was at boarding school on the coast of East Anglia. A splendid place, I'm sure, but by golly it wasn't half cold in winter. You had to be careful what you said to people, because if you made enemies they might come round and puncture your hot water bottle. During the really bad freeze of 1963 girls hung around the library begging for copies of the *Daily Telegraph* to stuff down the insides of their pyjama legs.

I don't know what other women remember about their schooldays—scoring the winning goal in the grudge match against St Monica's at hockey, perhaps, or fun filled midnight feasts when the dorm rippled with girlish laughter. I remember chilblains. Oh, I realise that, as medical events go, chilblains are pretty dull stuff. Unlike the birth of your firstborn, they do not make a good video with which to delight your friends and relations. However, for several years they dominated my life. The only available remedy seemed to be a thick greyish ointment which you had to smear all over your throbbing, itching feet before bedtime. I knew that I would never be able to have a sex life, for what man would want to snuggle up to a creature who had to live in a pool of grease all winter, like a confit de canard?

Not that we were encouraged to think about sex, anyway. One 40 minute slide show was all we received, delivered by the biology mistress, who, made dyslexic with embarrassment, got several of the slides upside down and in the wrong order. For some time afterwards I had a very bizarre idea of male anatomy.

Fortunately, we found out what we needed to know from the Ass Mats, who were usually young and pretty girls just out of nursery nurse college. The most scandalous was the rather inaptly named Miss Nunn, who used to answer all our questions about the *Kama Sutra* when she was meant to be taking lights out. It was a subject on which she had obviously had a certain amount of experience. Around midway through the summer term we noticed she had put on a lot of weight around the waist. Then one night she rushed out during supper and brought up her spam fritters in the head-mistress's rose garden, after which she was abruptly replaced by someone warty and elderly with a tight grey perm.

The Ass Mats were ruled by Sister, a spiky Latvian refugee who roamed the school sanatorium in a flapping white coat with keys jangling from her belt. Sister spoke a fierce but limited English. Instead of, for instance, saying, "In order to help your body fight this viral infection you should drink lots of water," she would bring her face very close to yours and shout, "Fluids plus, plus, plus!" She was so terrifying that girls would have died, almost literally, rather than get banged up in the san with her.

What never ceases to amaze me, though, is now healthy we have all turned out to be. Recently I went to an Old Girls day where my classmates, now approaching middle age, were to a woman bright of eye, steady of hand, and trim of ankle. When I think back to my schooldays I remember what I learnt about health. The best cure for chilblains is a centrally heated house. Spam fritters make you sick. And, unless you are an octopus, position 96 of the *Kama Sutra* is not a good idea.

AWAY FROM IT ALL

We have just had our annual summer holiday in Catalonia, where we stay in a house in the Spanish equivalent of National Trust land. Here amid the din of oleanders bursting into bloom we sit on the terrace enjoying our statutory alcoholic intake of 14 units, the difference being that in Spain this somehow seems to end up being per meal rather than per week. If we're bored there's always the flypast of swallows at six every night, and the lizard is good value, especially when it does its famous slalom from the patio light fitting into the geranium bed.

The suspicion that this is Arcadia is strengthened by the discovery that no fewer than three out of the seven adjacent holiday homes are occupied by doctors, who presumably know when they're on to a good thing when it comes to lowering the blood pressure and knitting up the ravelled sleeve of care.

Mind you, I always think that admitting you're a doctor on holiday is a mistake, especially if you speak English. Our national mistrust of foreign medics is so entrenched that the minute you let slip your calling the entire British contingent within a 10 mile radius will bring you their concussed children, their paella-ravaged digestive systems, their mosquito bites ("Are you absolutely certain it isn't skin cancer?"). Don't worry if you're a world famous neurosurgeon or a Harley Street gynaecologist. You won't be left out. We don't stand on ceremony here.

Being a journalist has its drawbacks—I am never able to slough off the memory of the all-in wrestler who threatened to find out my home address after I wrote about him in terms that caused offence—but so far no member of the public has approached me on a beach and said confidentially, "I say, I know you're on holiday but would you mind letting me have 800 words on what's wrong with British tennis by noon tomorrow?"

Doctors, on the other hand, are never allowed to be off duty. I don't know if Livingstone was a doctor of medicine but if so I expect the full unexpurgated text of Stanley's greeting was on the lines of, "Dr Livingstone, I presume? Look, I know you're meant to be getting away from it all but I'm having a spot of bother with the old waterworks, wonder if you'd mind checking me out, don't like the look of these local quacks at all."

19

Of course, once you experience the Spanish medical system you realise that there is no cause for alarm. When our then teenaged son fell of his bike and grazed his leg on a track used by sheep, we dragged him off for a tetanus shot to the nearest health centre where he was treated by a superbly competent young woman doctor who not only spoke excellent English but made Sophia Loren seem like Les Dawson in comparison.

Spanish pharmacists are also worth a visit. Their over the counter medicines are far more macho than their British counterparts. There is, for instance, a marvellously effective preparation for cleaning the scale off lavatory bowls which is on the banned list over here, probably because in sufficient quantities it is capable of dissolving a medium range jet. As in France, it is customary for some medicines to be taken in suppository form, and indeed Spanish pharmacies can supply a treatment for haemorrhoids which is reputed to be particularly soothing.

Some English friends of ours often take Spanish medicines home with them. One year they were having a relaxing lunchtime drink in the village square when a waiter came rushing out of the bar waving a telegram that had just arrived for them. Dry throated and white faced, they tore open the envelope to find out what disaster had befallen their house, their teenage children, the dog, the car. The message was signed, Grandma, and read DON'T FORGET THE BUM PASTILLES.

Bernard Dixon

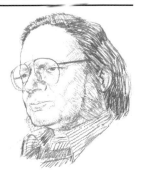

A LITTLE ELEMENTARY SCIENCE

R emember that business with a burning candle in a dish of water? You place a glass jar upside down over the candle and watch the water rise as the oxygen in the air is consumed and the flame dies away. You then measure the height of the water and show that it represents one fifth of the height of the jar. Whether as a classroom demonstration or a children's party trick, the experiment proves that oxygen comprises one fifth of the air we breathe.

Right? Well, maybe. But on the whole probably not. Forty years after querying the matter with an unhelpful science teacher (he told me not to be so silly, boy), I am still awaiting a convincing account of this deceptively simple diversion. The problem with the conventional explanation arises from that canny Italian lawyer turned physicist, Amedo Avogadro. A paper published by Avogadro in 1811 enshrined what is now a law that carries his name and that really messes up our tidy explanation of the candle experiment.

Avogadro's law states that equal volumes of different gases at the same temperature and pressure contain the same number of molecules. So what happens to the oxygen in the jar as the candle burns to extinction? Answer: it is converted into an equal volume of carbon dioxide. That stuff about one fifth of the air being "consumed" cannot be right. Indeed, one wonders why the water rises at all.

Maybe it does so because carbon dioxide is much more soluble, as compared with oxygen, in water? Not so. But there's another possibility. Perhaps some of the air bubbles away when it is warmed by the candle flame and expands accordingly, the remaining air contracting as it cools, sucking up water and producing an entirely bogus fifth? Not really—close observation shows no such bubbling.

Then there's the awkward fact that published descriptions of the experiment show that the water level rises not by a predictable fifth but by anything between 14% and 24%. To make matters worse, one of those reports shows that the candle invariably goes out when the oxygen content of the air falls from its original 21%, not to 0%, but to 14–16%.

Over the years I have heard many different explanations of this apparently trivial phenomenon. The most Byzantine came from a talented chemist whom I consulted with some diffidence, believing that he could put my mind at rest in a crisp sentence or two. Instead, he gave me a 15 minute lecture on the combustion products of candle wax, and insisted that somewhere therein lay the answer. But a week later he rang back to say that he was having second thoughts. I have not heard from him since.

The whole thing is reminiscent of the correspondence that once ran for many months in *New Scientist*, following a Nigerian student's claim that warm water could freeze more quickly than cold. The most striking aspect of that episode was the total confidence with which successive writers demonstrated, with a wide variety of arguments, that the student was wrong, or right, or indeed right and wrong according to circumstances.

Anyone with a crisp—and watertight—sentence or two?

APES AND ESSENCES

Observations of medical strategies in primitive human societies have provided many valuable insights—into indigenous drugs, for example. But what of instinctive or culturally transmitted knowledge about herbal remedies among wild animals, and especially primates? I have wondered about this possibility ever since reading of wild boars in India eating so called pigweed—a plant that is, apparently, of modest nutritional value but which contains agents effective against many pig-infesting helminths.

Now I see from a paper by Paul Newton of Wolfson College, Oxford, in the admirable *Trends in Ecology and Evolution* (vol 6, p 297) that animal pharmacy is indeed on a sound footing. Reviewing several recent pieces of research, Newton concludes that non-human primates have developed a particularly complex battery of herbal drugs. He believes that this could well comprise a neglected source of information regarding substances with potential for treating human disease too.

Just as striking as the evidence of primates ingesting plants for other than nutritional purposes is their mode of use. One field observation is that of the "non-chewing" technique first recorded among wild chimpanzees at Gombe in Tanzania. While Gombe's chimps eat leaves in general mostly during the afternoons, they consume *Aspilia* leaves in the morning only. The other difference is that instead of chomping this shrub into fragments they simply massage blades between the tongue and buccal surface and then swallow them whole. They also use *Aspilia* leaves half as quickly as when foraging generally.

As Newton points out, the chimp's non-chewing technique, puzzling at first, is actually very similar to the buccal and sub-lingual administration of drugs such as glyceryl trinitrate in human medicine. Its use by Tanzanian chimpanzees may well be related to the presence in *Aspilia* leaves of high concentrations of thiarubrine, a potent destroyer of bacteria, fungi, and nematodes. Recent reports indicate that chimps adopt the same method when ingesting leaves of *Lippia*, which also provides an African folk medicine taken for malaria and dysentery. There is even one published description of a lethargic and anorexic female, thought to be suffering from gastrointestinal symptoms, who was sucking bitter juice from the shoot pith of *Vernonia amyglalina*—a bush widely used to treat intestinal disorders in both humans and livestock.

Does self prescribing by chimpanzees—the result of natural selection after countless trials and errors—point to an untapped reservoir of medicinal information relevant to the human pharmacopoeia? I wonder.

BERNARD DIXON

ELIMINATING DISEASE

I see that the World Health Organisation, which announced the global eradication of smallpox in 1979, is boldly forecasting that a second disease-causing organism is likely to become little more than a grim historical memory. The WHO believes that *Dracunculus medinensis*, the agent of guinea worm disease, is now destined to be wiped from the face of the earth. After dramatic successes in reducing the toll of human suffering caused by this water borne malady in India, Pakistan, and sub-Saharan Africa, total global eradication is now considered achievable by 1995.

A note of caution may be in order, however. This is to belittle neither WHO's achievement so far, nor its hope for the future, but simply to underline the size of the problems still to be overcome. We should remember that the smallpox virus was an exceptionally vulnerable target for obliteration. It has no reservoir other than humans, and it does not alter its antigenic clothing by mutating or swapping fragments of DNA. Its transmission can be blocked as a result of the solid, long lasting immunity induced by immunisation with vaccinia.

Many other pathogens have proved much more difficult to eradicate. Some are ruled out by their complexities of life cycles involving secondary hosts, or by inadequate immunity after vaccination. In other cases the obstacle is the capacity of the organism to develop resistance to drugs, or the resourcefulness of its vector in becoming insensitive to insecticides. The malarial parasite illustrates every one of these difficulties and is thus likely to be with us for a very long time.

Yet even those viruses that did once seem threatened by worldwide elimination now seem less promising candidates. With poliomyelitis there are unresolved worries over the sporadic appearance of cases caused by virus strains derived from the vaccine itself. Measles, too, may be wiped out in time, though optimism based on its eradication from several states in the United States during the 1970s is now thought to have been premature. In these and other cases the task of delivering vaccines to the requisite number of people over the right period of time remains formidable.

Until WHO's recent announcement about guinea worm disease, the condition most discussed as next in line for global elimination was not a human disease at all but a bovine infection, rinderpest. Long since exterminated in Europe, rinderpest is now largely confined to equatorial Africa, the Middle East, and south Asia. Progress, however, has not been uniformly smooth. While transmission of the causative virus can be blocked by vaccination, political actions have often hindered rather than promoted immunisation campaigns.

In the case of guinea worm disease, eradication efforts are based not on immunisation but on tactics such as boiling drinking water and filtering it to remove the larvae of cyclops, the minute crustacean that carries *Dracunculus*. These simple measures have reduced the total of cases from 10 million during the 1980s to under three million today. The same rate of progress could indeed see the global task completed by the WHO's target date of 1995. Let us hope that politics promote, rather than impede, the appropriate logistics.

LYME AND THE LAYPERSON

" These lay pressures groups are interfering with research. . . . There is science and there is non-science, and non-science doesn't belong at a scientific meeting."

Such was the angry reaction of Durland Fish of New York Medical College in Valhalla, speaking as a member of the programme committee for the fifth international conference on Lyme borreliosis, held recently in Arlington, Virginia. His irritation, according to a report in *Science* (1992; **256**:1384), followed the reinstatement of several papers originally rejected by the committee as not meeting the conventional standards of peer review. Written by non-academic clinicians, the papers were put back on the agenda largely as a result of pressure from patient support groups. Principal issues at stake included the question of whether patients described in the controversial reports were really suffering from Lyme disease (now, apparently, an over diagnosed condition in the United States) and whether they were receiving valid treatments.

Perhaps Fish is right. Perhaps not. But the incident brings vividly to mind the not dissimilar circumstances under which Lyme disease itself came to public prominence for the first time. They deserve to be rememberred now, and indeed on all occasions when the scientific establishment, with its quite proper regard for rigour in the assessment of evidence, has to respond to challenges that can all too readily be dismissed as insubstantial, wacky, or beyond the pale.

Back in 1975, in Connecticut, a mother drew the attention of state health department officials to the fact that no fewer than 12 children in one village, Old Lyme, were suffering from an illness that had been diagnosed as juvenile rheumatoid arthritis. Another woman went to the Yale rheumatology clinic with news of an alleged "epidemic" of arthritis in her family. There were observations which the community's health surveillance machinery had totally missed. To some officials they sounded distinctly weird. Who had ever heard of an epidemic of arthritis?

Gradually, a group of concerned parents in Old Lyme came together and began to lobby for the mystery to be investigated. One research group, at Yale, did take it seriously and started to monitor what was happening. By 1977 they had become convinced that there was indeed an outbreak, of what later became known as Lyme arthritis. As well as causing aching joints, this strange condition had two major characteristics. It tended to begin in summer, and it appeared among children or adults several weeks after they had acquired an unusual type of papule on the skin.

The first real clue to the cause of the condition came when one patient recalled having been bitten by a tick at the site of the papule. Detective work then led from serology to the isolation of the causative spirochaete from the tick. Clever stuff. Yet a major lesson from this episode was that public, rather than professional, disquiet brought the problem to light in the first place.

Twenty years ago Dr Fish would have raised little or no dissent among his peers for dismissing epidemic arthritis as non-science. But he would have been wrong, wouldn't he?

DON'T EXPORT
MISTRUST

The good news at Christmas for *Nature* readers was of some stunning results from the first large scale field trial of a genetically engineered vaccine against rabies. Baits containing a hybrid vaccinia-rabies virus, dropped by helicopter over large areas of southern Belgium, induced immunity to the disease in more than 80% of foxes sampled later. The incidence of rabies declined rapidly during the trial and no cases have been reported since, either in foxes or in domestic animals. Four cheers for recombinant DNA technology.

Future exercises in the release of genetically engineered microbes into the environment are unlikely to proceed so smoothly. Belgium is one of the few countries in Europe where the deliberate dissemination of such organisms has not attracted spirited opposition from activist groups. Elsewhere, particularly in the former West Germany, the past five years have seen fierce antagonism towards the idea that viruses and bacteria carrying "foreign" genes can be safely released—whether to promote soil fertility, to prevent insect attacks on plants, or to induce immunity in humans and other animals. Scientists have been vilified in Holland, petunia patches picketed in Cologne.

The dreadful convulsions of rabies are, of course, a shrewd target through which to publicise the beneficence of this new technology. Few fairminded bystanders would quibble at the motives behind such an achievement. The practicalities are a different matter, however, and critics will go on fighting against research which they believe (whether through ignorance or knowledge) to be inherently unsafe. Scientists and companies developing genetically modified organisms for medical, veterinary, and agricultural purposes need to work hard to foster public trust.

What they should *not* do is to opt out by taking their projects to the other side of the world, where regulations are minimal and antiscience campaigners unknown. There are, unfortunately, signs that this could happen. At least two German firms, BASF and Hoechst, have chosen to locate new recombinant DNA facilities abroad rather than in their own country, because of anxieties concerning overregulation. Hoechst's decision followed a particularly frustrating episode when local lobbyists delayed by three

27

years the opening of a new plant for genetically engineered insulin near Frankfurt. Representatives of Sandoz and other companies have also voiced growing concerns about a climate of public apprehension and unduly severe controls over biotechnology in Europe.

The only concrete instance thus far of a Western nation going elsewhere to conduct field work with a genetically engineered organism has been that of the Philadelphia based Wistar Institute carrying out studies with a recombinant rabies vaccine in Argentina, allegedly in contravention of that country's laws on the importation of "exotic" micro-organisms. One hopes that the furious reaction to this event (both by Argentinian scientists and by critics abroad) will persuade other groups that the export of novel technology is not the answer to their dilemma. The one sure consequence of such a policy would be to signal that such work really is inherently hazardous. All the signs now are that this is simply not true.

GUNPOWDER AND GAMMA RAYS

Even to an innocent 9 year old, asking a pharmacist for the constituents of gunpowder seemed a risky thing to do. So I set out to make the request seem more authoritative by typing out the list—saltpetre, charcoal, and flowers of sulphur—on a borrowed typewriter with a new ribbon and good quality paper. I then signed my "prescription" and added the date at the bottom. It was an impressive document, specifying the correct proportions of the desired ingredients.

Though well prepared in this way, it was with a mixture of confidence and apprehension that I opened the door of the local pharmacy and approached the counter. I expected to be served by the shop assistant (a neighbour, as it happened) but instead the rather forbidding Mr Norman Willis MPS stepped forward from his gloomy dispensary. He perused my sheet of paper, looked out into the street, glowered at me for what felt like several hours, and then turned on his heel and walked away without a word.

A few minutes later Mr Willis returned, with a face like thunder. He gave me an angry glance, grunted, and put something on the counter. I looked down, but he immediately retrieved the package and placed a warning hand on my arm. "Now look here laddie," he said. "If you ever come in here again, you'll not be served if you forget to close that door."

Attitudes have certainly changed, from an age when a small boy could make bombs in the garden shed to the modern era of ultra safety in which chemistry sets contain nothing more exciting than logwood chips and filter paper. From time to time one is reminded of those earlier, more robust days with such force that their insouciance seems hardly credible. A good example is to be found in an article by Ray Harrop and colleagues in that constantly absorbing journal, *Chemistry in Britain* (1992; **28**:399). It describes a do it yourself radiotherapy kit, sold during the 1930s, called the Qray Electro-Radioactive Dry Compress.

A canvas case containing a heating element and pitchblende (the radioactive ore from which the Curies extracted radium), the device was marketed as "a relief for rheumatism, sciatica, invaluable for pneumonia and bronchial complaints." A Professor Singer MD, chief medical officer at the Rudolfsiftung Hospital in Vienna, had endorsed the Qray, whose rays were said to "travel at 186,000 miles a second, penetrate the epidermidis and reach the nerve endings through the blood stream."

In the light of modern knowledge, use of a device of this sort sounds quite terrifying. Tests by Harrop and his coauthors indicate that the Qray delivered in just one hour more than a tenth of today's recommended maximum dose for the general population over an entire year. More difficult to fathom is why the machine was on sale a decade after the first evidence that gamma rays from radioactive elements could damage and destroy red blood cells. And there's an even more perplexing problem. Why was this extraordinary piece of equipment, obtained through a local environmental health officer from the house of a lady recently deceased, carrying a modern 13 amp plug?

Colin Douglas

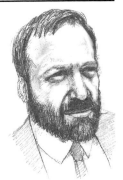

THE DETACHED
RETINUE
SYNDROME

Bismarck, it is said, decided upon 65 as the standard retirement age in order to rid himself at a stroke of a host of vexatious functionaries in Berlin. Retirement at 65 proved to be one of Germany's earliest export successes. It was adopted widely in the Western world, is criticised for its rigidity, but is still broadly enforced. In medicine, and particularly in academic medicine, it sometimes poses problems.

The profession of medicine is competitive and no less so in its higher reaches. The drive for power (and, it goes without saying, for higher standards in research, teaching, and clinical service) does not reliably disappear on the 65th birthday, or even at the end of the month or academic term within which that anniversary falls. It follows that the most senior figures in the profession approach retirement with feelings ranging from relief through contentment and bewilderment to frank denial.

Those whose responses are in the most negative categories are more at risk. Such skills, influence, and authority as they have nurtured carefully or indeed obsessively over the years are suddenly devalued, and a variety of strategies may be adopted to minimise the impact of their loss. Men—and it is seen for the moment predominantly as a male problem, data on women being, for whatever reasons, exiguous—at whose whim jobs, money, rewards, and retributions were once instantly dispensed suddenly find themselves wondering how to get a letter typed. Responses

31

vary. Recognition of patterns of dysfunctional behaviour following loss of staff and status forms the basis of diagnosis of the detached retinue syndrome (DRS).

Happy the head of department whose predecessor has retired, for family reasons, to Tasmania. He need not fear that slow, familiar footstep on the stair; that inquiry about how—in general or in particular—things are going; that casual request that some distinguished foreigners (now of course also retired) be accommodated with a three week programme of departmental activities in which the predecessor himself would be happy to play a modest part. Former junior colleagues are also vulnerable. They find their age and status mysteriously frozen in time, and it is a dubious tribute to their conditioning that, despite still being treated as senior house officers, greying mid-lifers can remain gracious.

Treatment is unsatisfactory. A radical surgical approach is poorly tolerated. For established DRS palliation remains the best option, with the royal colleges providing extensive facilities for day (and in some cases evening) respite care. Otherwise well elderly DRS sufferers, many of them taking advantage of pensioners' subsidised travel, can be accommodated in harmless diversional activities such as committees, working groups, advisory bodies, and participation in examinations for higher degrees.

The small minority of severe DRS cases offers the greatest challenge. For those from whom the most serious disruption can be anticipated there is a costly but helpful resource at present available only in central London. With good access for the disabled, copious toilet facilities, subsidised catering, and unrivalled peer support, it offers excellent extended care—but for very limited numbers. Applications (enclose SAE) should be made direct to the House of Lords, London SW1A 0PW. Sadly, as is so often the case with public sector provisions for the elderly, there is a long waiting list.

WITH CONTENTS

R ESIDENTIAL HOME FOR THE ELDERLY, REGISTERED FOR FIFTEEN. FOR SALE AS GOING CONCERN. The smart green and white sign at the gate puts much else to shame: lawns are neglected and the gravel drive is carpeted with worn grass. The house itself is a substantial century old Graeco-Caledonian villa. To one side it has sprouted at some time within the past 30 years a low extension the roughcast exterior of which is now wearing less well than the original's Craigleith stone. The doorbell works.

In the lounge are fifteen old ladies variously slumped on chairs and sofas. The air is dead and musty, the room silent. One old lady gets up and moves across to a sofa where another lies, her skirt up past her knees. The skirt is rearranged and the silent helper returns to her seat. Are male visitors unusual, perhaps unwelcome?

In the hall again, it is possible to ask questions. Yes, more than half the ladies are incontinent and rather more need help to walk. And the social work department is getting more and more particular about space, toilets, and fire safety. A sixteenth old lady shuffles past. That raises questions, but my guide explains that she is in fact the live-in cook and housekeeper.

The proprietor is unavailable. The tour goes on. Big Victorian ground floor rooms have been cubicalised into little pink and white hutches a bed and a half long, a bed wide. Photographs, hair-brushes, books, and slippers signify individuals. There is a shower, but the ladies don't like it.

Up a once grand staircase there are more bedrooms, some quite pleasant, others so cramped as to prompt more unsolicited information about the views of the social work department. One old lady has on a shelf the complete works of Alistair MacLean in paperback. Some of them are great readers, I am informed. No one in the lounge had been reading.

My guide explains a little more. Some of the ladies have visitors, others are so old that everybody's dead. Five years ago it wasn't too bad, but it's getting heavier all the time now. Fewer and fewer can walk by themselves and there isn't one that can get up the stairs without a hand. And of course the Department of Social Security supplement doesn't cover things these days, even though it's the social work department that's making it harder all the time.

The official story is that the proprietor has simply decided to retire, taking with him the live-in cook-housekeeper. In the mixed economy of health and social care a small business is struggling. The market is uncertain just now, because of interest rates and because no one knows what the effects of changes in the funding of care will be. Offers are invited but the FOR SALE board outside has been there for some weeks.

I thank my guide and we make our way downstairs again. On the walls of the stairwell hang dozens of decorative plates: blue and white Delft; garish red and gilt mementoes of forgotten Scottish resorts; fiords, cathedrals, tartans, and the inevitable portrait of the national bard with his old fashioned Elvis Presley sideburns. At eye level on the turn of the stair is a small white plate with a gilt rim and a gilt injunction in inch high copperplate: GOD BLESS OUR HOME.

PATRONAGE

A few years ago the editor of Another Leading Medical Journal asked me to write an editorial about the role of patronage in medicine. Given a generous deadline I read the scanty and rather cryptic literature on the subject, began to work, but then worried that the editorial would have been a model of worst editorialising practice; on the one hand agonising about the evidence, on the other failing miserably to make up its mind.

I am still uncertain about patronage in medicine and regret that ED, *ALMJ* is still waiting for his piece. I am, however, now in a position to explain what went wrong. Either he should have asked someone considerably younger (and preferably a woman), so that the whole system could have been exposed for the self serving hypocrisy and scandal it undoubtedly is and both the profession and the public at large thus informed of a cosy little conspiracy—sexist, racist, and old school tieist—that dispenses lifelong injustice in the guise of openly contested appointments. Alternatively, he could have asked someone a good deal more senior, who could have pontificated serenely from a lifetime's experience of the subtle appraisal of the magnitude of factors—technical, scientific, and personal—that have to be taken into account in maintaining the excellence and indeed the stability and much valued public esteem of our most ancient of professions—with results which, on the whole, reflect most creditably on all concerned.

The trouble, of course, is that I am as puzzled about patronage as almost everyone else in the middle reaches of the trade. On the one hand early medical life is a complex and uncertain business and there are times when it seems a duty and even a privilege to help a promising young doctor along the way with a supporting telephone call or a quiet word somewhere. On the other the systematic abuse of similar tactics by colleagues perhaps considerably more influential than oneself can often lead to the most flagrant injustice.

Whatever doubts there are about the morality of it all, patronage influences progress. We know people—from school, from medical school, from firms and departments. We arrange outselves into interest groups, broadly self perpetuating, composed of benefactors and beneficiaries, and that is the substance of most patronage in medicine. It undoubtedly exists, but that is not to say that it exists for everyone. Perhaps the most powerful but least discussed influence on the careers of young women in hospital medicine is the failure of older men to look after them. It is true that women's careers are more likely to be disrupted by their marrying, moving, and multiplying, but they could survive all that a good deal better if, like their male compeers, they became, by invitation and acceptance, the courteous and grateful adherents of someone in a position to help them until such time as they no longer needed that kind of help and could begin to dispense it themselves.

Generally speaking, women don't do things like that; but it is worth speculating on what might happen if they did. Think of a mafia run by a couple of dozen steely haired dames in teaching hospitals; a mysterious mechanism for sidelining perfectly adequate male candidates whose only shortcoming is that they happen to be men; a quiet but pervasive sisterhood sufficiently indefinable to defy confrontation but relentlessly effective in placing its chosen candidates year after year. Of course it's absurd, unthinkable, even outrageous. But then matronage would be, wouldn't it?

COLIN DOUGLAS

HEALTH PREVENTION IN SCOTLAND

Ben Starav is a remote and serious hill of 1078 metres, its northern ridge—a dreary slog from sea level at the foot of Glen Etive—seemingly deserted this Sunday morning. Odd therefore that at about 500 metres a breeze brings the voices of unseen fellow climbers in leisured conversation, odder still that it also carries unmistakable cigarette smoke.

We reach the cairn in fair time. There is no view, only a thin cold mist. We pause long enough for some coffee, not long enough to seize up, and just as we have set off on the jagged ridge westward two others arrive: middle aged men moving fast over the heaped boulders of the summit.

The mist thickens briefly to rain then clears long enough to allow a couple of compass fixes on summits that do not seem to be in the right place. Not to worry: the map is unequivocal, the path narrow but unmistakable, with nowhere to go other than along a spiked grey dragon's back veined here and there with quartz. Stags roar unseen in the glens below.

The ridge broadens and Glas Beinn Mhor looms ahead. On its summit, three and a half hours from the car, we stop and break out lunch. From the mist behind come the other two. They seem pleased to see us. "We thought we'd lost you just back there."

Organised Gortex-clad Munro-baggers don't say things like that, nor do survivors from the previous generation of hill walkers, the ones with sticks and long green stockings. These men are neither. It transpires that they have no map or compass, instead only a smudged photocopy of a page with notes and a rough sketch, from a book that specifically warns readers against taking to the hills with that alone. From half way up the northern ridge of Starav they have been using us as a kind of mobile sign post, one that must have kept disappearing into the mist.

They were out drinking until two this morning. Their boots are of the kind immediately seized upon by fatal accident inquiries. They shiver in light jerkins and have not brought enough to eat. They are grateful for a couple of tuna sandwiches and, perhaps because we are vaguely middle class, touchingly mistake them for salmon. In return they offer cigarettes around but do not seem offended when we decline them.

Sitting on boulders in the mist we talk at leisure. They come from near Stirling and work in a mysteriously surviving factory there. As a doctor I am offered details of hangovers, bronchitis, ulcer surgery, Zantac, Brufen, and sciatica. Sciatica? On Glas Beinn Mhor? "It's not too bad if you just keep walking. But maybe if you've got something for blisters. . . ."

I dispense Elastoplast, a lot of it, because the patient's socks are thin nylon. Eventually they stub out their cigarettes, cough a bit more, and we all set off. On the way down they make better speed than we do. The mist clears and we last see them waving farewell from far below.

Not a great place for health education, Scotland. At least not yet. But you can see right away where we get our world class, slightly suicidal infantrymen from.

TILL RETIREMENT DO YOU PART

"May we have the first candidate, please?" A solemn ritual, repeated with minor variations hundreds of times a year throughout the health service, has begun. On a side table are cups, saucers, and a plate of biscuits. Late in the afternoon tea leaves will be read, a junior hospital doctor made senior, a career remuneration of well over £1 million at today's rates allotted, a colleague appointed. It is a serious matter. We must all try to stay awake.

Traditionally the ones most likely to stay awake are the candidates and those with whom the appointee will work for the foreseeable future. The less involved do well at first but attention soon wanders—the candidate deals politely with the same question twice in five minutes—and eyelids begin to droop. Looking round the pictures helps, as does taking copious notes.

The national panellists are on prickly form. My colleague and I, the two most involved, listen to them, aware that they can make choices difficult but not impossible. They are concerned. We are involved. They claim their expenses and go. We stay, to embark with someone on a relationship much less dissoluble than marriage. Others may doze, roused in turn to take up the questioning. Like the succession of candidates appearing at the uncomfortable end of the table, my colleague and I stay awake.

The candidates are courteous and forbearing. They take our questions—variously probing, banal, self important, repetitive, and sometimes not questions at all—and make the best of them, talking with knowledge and feeling about the specialty and its future. They play gently to our foibles but do not talk down to us. Whatever they may say about us before and after, their comportment here is charm itself. One would almost think their lives depended on it.

Two hours pass slowly. No one actually yawns, but a senior figure with vast experience of these affairs seems to take the view that it is better to be well rested for the discussion. Perhaps he's right. The number of cups, saucers, and biscuits has been calculated precisely. When I was appointed the windows were clean, but that was a long time ago. At 4.20 pm tea is served.

"An outstanding field of candidates. . . ." We proceed to the measuring out of lives with NHS teaspoons, and the senior figure is suddenly awake and effective. Had he been listening all the time? And the man who asked exactly the same three questions four times running now says little. The candidates had to take him seriously; the committee might not. The national panellists unbend fractionally. Discussion is at first general then quite swiftly focused. The job, the cumulative million plus, the near indissoluble relationship is no longer anyone's. An appointment is about to be made.

There is of course no explicit right of sitting consultants to choose their colleagues. Why should there be? ("But we've *always* been a firm of diligent bores/clubbable commercial rogues/violently obsessional workaholics, etc, etc.") But as the discussion reaches its final stages there is detectable tactful awareness on the part of those who can walk away from the decision for the feelings of those who can't. There is no serious disagreement. When recalled to the committee room with its dirty windows the successful candidate seems pleased too. Perhaps she feels she could work with us.

SOLDIERING ON

The casualty lies as he fell, a Sunday morning painter happy on a ladder until moments ago. Unconscious now, supine and grunting for breath, with blood seeping from his left thigh and a huge contusion on his forehead, he poses several problems. Someone lifts his jaw forward. That seems to help.

He breathes more easily but remains unresponsive. The bulging, bleeding thigh might be his worst injury but there are others: an obvious compound tibial fracture on the right, plus a wrist that hardly matters. Slowly his eyes open. That makes it all a bit easier.

Yes, he can feel that, and that. But not that. No, his legs don't hurt at all, in fact he can't feel anything below his waist. He closes his eyes again and sighs. Gently we straighten his left leg. He feels no pain. Perhaps someone should phone for an ambulance now. Odd that no one thought of that, but at least we can give them a clear idea of what they'll find. "Good," says our crisp Glaswegian instructress. "And just one other point. Tell them where you are. Ambulance men are quite particular about that." The casualty smiles.

Except for him, everyone is in uniform and wears a Haig Fund poppy. Naval and army reservist medical officers, we are learning trauma life support, British Army style, over a weekend in a vast, bleak, and deserted northern garrison. Our Armistice Sunday began at 8 am with a debriefing on a paper triage exercise, a homely matter of half a dozen civilian road traffic casualties. By 10 we had covered spinal injuries and burns, and towards 11 we are grappling with a triage exercise far fiercer though mercifully still on paper: a vignette from a European land battle that the Russians seem to be winning.

They have crossed the Weser and shot up one of our forward positions. Nine wounded men, variously blasted, burned, and bleeding, arrive at our paper field ambulance; with not much time and too little transport back, difficult decisions must be made.

All over the country other people wearing poppies gather round war memorials. Stuck in our chilly classroom we ponder and scribble, examinees in heavy duty first aid and the art of rationing amid the unrationed carnage of war. There are rules and we know them. Imagination does not help. Sympathy does. This one will die: soon, comfortably, and without the folly of another journey. Move him out into the sun. Next please.

Thirty minutes of that, a 50 question multiple choice question-naire, and it is all over. By 12.30 we are back in the mess. Life has appeared in Catterick, in the form of officers, their ladies, and children—all on their best after-church behaviour—gathering for the traditional Armistice Sunday drinks and lunch. We are out of place. Transient, anomalous in uniform, eager to be off, and perhaps still too close to what we have been learning about to enjoy the party, we decide to eat straight away.

Wherever the union jack still flies Armistice Sunday lunch is always curry, a legacy of empire done to traditional military recipes few restaurateurs would copy. We eat quickly, almost guiltily, at a table under a mysterious picture of haggard French infantrymen retreating from Moscow. Our Russians are not coming, but we have learnt a lot. Soon we will be civilians again, driving home through the sad shires. No one has a second helping.

VISITORS

Down the years our little academic department has endured with fortitude an inevitable consequence of its modest repu-tation in rather a thin specialty: we are more visited against than visiting.

To say that is not to complain about our many and various guests. They are generally interested, polite, grateful, and keen to reciprocate our hospitality. ("Any time you're in Kalamazoo you'll drop by, wontcha, huh? Great.") Some come alone; some in droves with translators and buses, like package tours. Some come with expectations so high that we can only disappoint them. Some fit us in, for tax reasons, between ancestor hunts in the graveyards of Connemara and culture splurges at your wonderful Eden-burg Festival.

Some seem intent on writing down everything we say, as though our specialty were a culture dying in the hands of a dwindling band of preliterate aborigines. Others seem to think it is less trouble for us if they talk all the time, usually about how they do it at home. A few sad souls appear to have been sent off by their departments to travel the world as some kind of penance or punishment, so that we worry about what they might find when they get back.

There are occasional surprises. Once a distinguished Third World physician arrived and, having completed the basic tour, expressed an interest in a service development in which we take some pride. Arrangements were made. After two and a half hours of introductory explanation, ward visits, and multidisciplinary case conferences through which he had sat solemn, silent, and evidently engrossed, I asked him if he had any questions. He brightened up a lot. "Yes, yes," he said. "Where please can I buy some coat hangers?"

Next day I gave him some of the wire ones that proliferate mysteriously in all middle class wardrobes. Recently I thought of him again. Everything had changed. I was a visitor, living out of a suitcase in a strange land with more weather than climate, visiting a busy academic unit and trying, within the limits of language, to discern the subtleties of complex specialty arrangements amid a system of health care quite different from our own. My sympathy for the brave souls who visit our department had increased enormously. I suppose I knew what it felt like.

Sitting in the offices of a variety of busy people I wondered again and again what they might be doing if they were not looking after me. My respect for their tolerance of my total inability to speak their language knows no bounds. For them to speak English was only a minor chore, but it visibly deprived them of many of the little things—nuances, idioms, jokes—that go to make professional contacts rewarding and relaxing. They did valiantly and I am eternally in their debt.

I learnt a lot and I hope I did not cause them too much inconvenience. They were informative, cheerful, kind, and helpful when I felt vulnerable and burdensome and when they were undoubtedly busy. If ever any of them are in Edinburgh I sincerely hope they'll drop by. And in case you ever need to know, the Swedish for coat hanger is "klädehangäre."

NOTHING SERIOUS

The dual carriageway ends in a pool of sodium light at a roundabout. Thirty yards short of that a car, its hazard lights flashing, sits awkwardly astride the kerb.

Ahead of it a woman and a small child stand on the rough grass holding hands and looking round.

To stop or not? I am not in a hurry, but I am no mechanic either. Difficult. The road is a quiet one: no house in view and miles from any town or village. Difficult, because of a number of unplesant cases, but more difficult not to stop. I pull over 20 yards ahead of the car, a newish, mid-size Peugeot with a personalised registration number.

An unaccompanied male stranger, bearded and tieless, has stopped. How will that seem to them? I walk towards them but do not hurry. Another car passes. What might its occupants think, if indeed they notice? And is there even the faintest possibility that the next car to come along that quiet country road might shriek to a halt and disgorge three or four militant feminists wielding crowbars and not asking questions?

Two more cars pass in quick succession and neither stops. As I approach the pair standing in front of the Peugeot they do not seem alarmed. The woman is short and slight, pale under the sodium light. She is dressed in a track suit as is the child, a boy of about 5. He looks up and smiles, still holding his mother's hand. Or is he?

He is not holding her hand. He is holding the sleeve of her track suit. She has no hand and no arm either, left or right. She has scarcely any shoulders. "It's nothing serious," she tells me when I ask. "Just a hub cap. I heard the bang and saw it in the mirror." She smiles too. "But it was a long way to come back for it because of the dual carriageway."

They have found the hub cap. It is lying on the grass verge but they seem to have got stuck at that stage. I retrieve it and try to put it back where it belongs, on the front nearside wheel. There are problems. In the dark the spring catches are fiddly. Despite my best efforts it sits precariously. I am no mechanic.

So we decide they'll just take it home and her husband will see to it. They don't have far to go. The little boy is ordered into the back of the car, the hub cap placed on the floor at his feet. For a moment we chat, strangers in the night. I ask if she'll manage. She will. Of course she will, because everything was fine until the hub cap came off, but perhaps because I've helped a little she does not resent my curiosity. Thalidomide? Yes. The car, automatic gearbox apart, is ordinary and unmodified. I am still curious. She shrugs with her eyebrows. "I drive with my feet."

She thanks me and goes round to the driver's door, flips it open and hops in. I get back into my car and sit for a while, hazard lights ticking, still a sentry of some kind until they rejoin the safety of anonymous night traffic. The Peugeot lumbers off the verge behind, gathers speed and passes me. Its driver smiles again and waves: a cheerful left foot.

James Owen Drife

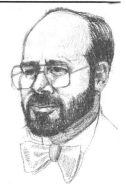

OPERATION NOTES

Operating today. ?Time to write article between cases. ?Why surgeons always write notes in telegraphese with no auxiliary verbs. Save time, perhaps. ?Why hospital notes always put question mark at *beginning* of sentence, not end. Complete mystery. Perhaps all hospitals originally staffed by Spaniards.

Surgeons and playwrights only people who work in pyjamas. But playwrights' pyjamas fit, I bet. Surgeons' not fit. Hospital laundry think surgical teams either Harlem Globetrotters or Seven Dwarfs. ?Why some surgical pyjamas have flies. Unnecessary—surgeons oliguric while operating. ?Deliberate insult by sewing room—flies only 1 cm diameter.

Furthermore, flies permanently open. Doctor's dilemma: ?ignore flies—risk upsetting student nurses (worse, amusing them); ?seal with sticking plaster—but pink too conspicuous, draw glances. Mind you, nurses use sticking plaster on theatre dresses—otherwise spectacular decolletage, surgeons distracted, patient at risk.

Watch out, thief about in changing room. Pyjama pocket not big enough bleep, watch, pen, chequebook, credit cards, filofax. Find locker with key. Key disappear hole in pocket damn blast, tie round neck on gauze bandage.

Where in blazes boots with name on? Forced wear clogs marked "student." Athlete's foot for sure. Clomp around taking surreptitious look everyone's heels. If catch student with consultant boots, have guts garters.

Surgical hats all disposable nowadays. High quality paper. "Made in Texas," says box, "assembled in Mexico." Mind

45

boggles. Paper hat traffic across Rio Grande, then transatlantic shipment—rum, molasses, paper hats. ?Why NHS choose Mexican hats. ?DoH worldwide hatfinding tour: find perfect hat—meet British Standard, not disintegrate midway through operation.

Flight of fancy. Hat trials in England and Mexico. Final test— hot lights, really incompetent surgeon, bathed in sweat throughout operation. Wonder why hats necessary anyway: most surgeons balding—in distinguished sort of way.

Scrub up now. Nailbrushes individually wrapped. Impossible open plastic packaging. Not allowed use teeth. Brushes made in Europe: multilingual instructions all over box. Now know how say "fingernails" eight languages. English, French, German, Spanish, er, Italian. . . . No, Italian, Spanish. ?Which one Norwegian.

Never managed get hang elbow taps. ?Left cold, right hot. ?Inwards off, outwards on. ?Other way round. Every hospital different. Sometimes think plumber visit weekly, change round. Three minutes later temperature just right, then houseman finish at other end, turn off her taps with flourish, surgeon utter silent scream.

Teach student scrubbing. Drop towel, Mr Smith. No, just *drop* it. Yes, on floor. ?Where else. Give me strength God. Thought sterile technique primordial instinct—like fear, rage. Forgot has to be learned.

Hate disposable gowns. Even higher quality paper. Cannot believe cheaper than laundry. Rio Grande long way off, heaven's sake. ?Why so cheap: ?nearer rainforest, ?cheap labour. Pity Mexican peasant—assemble hats all day, wife in cardboard city, dozen bambinos. And probably illiterate, poor thing.

ARE BREASTS REDUNDANT ORGANS?

Sometimes when I'm lecturing I point out how easy it would be to abolish breast cancer. My suggestion tends to outrage the men in the audience and I have to reassure them that my proposition is philosophical, not practical. Women listeners, however, usually react more thoughtfully.

Breast cancer becomes more common with age and will eventually affect at least one in 17 women in Britain. Screening may improve survival rates but does not aim at abolishing the disease altogether. The way to eradicate breast cancer is to remove the breasts before the cancer develops. The age at which she has the operation may be left to the woman. With the insertion of implants it could be carried out at any age, but the sensible option would be prophylactic mastectomy either at the completion of her family or at the menopause.

My suggestion is so shocking that I am beginning to lose my nerve as I type this. Why? The reason lies in the emotional importance not of the milk glands but of the fat that surrounds them. It is this fat that swells at puberty and makes a girl realise she is a woman. The fat has nothing to do with lactation but is a sexual signal, like the chimpanzee's swollen perineum. Men respond because they are programmed to do so, not because of cultural influences.

We hate to think that we are affected by instinct. Like hypnotists' victims we rationalise our reactions, but our feelings about breasts are far from logical. Women blame men for bad attitudes but the breast is much more important psychologically to women than to men. For a woman it is the main symbol of her femininity, and this is why she wants to retain it long after she has attracted a mate.

Even when a breast turns malignant a woman often wants to keep it. This is hardly rational. Many women in Britain undergo hysterectomy and few of them feel they are losing their femininity, but both sexes see mastectomy as unacceptably mutilating. Rationally, prophylactic mastectomy involves nothing more than excising a redundant gland and a pad of fat. Society should not deny this option to women, particularly those with a family history of breast cancer.

You can see, can't you, why my lecture upsets people. Men ask how I would like to be castrated, and look as if they mean this as a practical, not a philosophical, proposition. The analogy is inaccurate because, unlike the testis, the breast at 50 has no function apart from its psychological one. I refer questioners to my own secondary sexual characteristics and point out that if my beard had a 6% chance of turning malignant I would shave it off.

The audience eyes me warily, no doubt feeling there is something weird about a man who talks about removing normal breasts. They may be right. Perhaps all this is a distorted grief reaction to the deaths, over the years, of relatives, friends, and colleagues, killed painfully by glands they didn't need.

BREASTS AND THE MEDIA

The first hint of trouble came on Maundy Thursday. A reporter phoned, sounding excited. "Has anyone else rung?" "No." "They will," she replied. The *BMJ* had appeared with my "philosophical proposition" that prophylactic mastectomy could prevent cancer.

Good Friday's front page had accurate but highly selective quotes, and added that a London colleague thought my article "offensive." (The reporter had sent him a copy by fax.) Now the first papers had a controversy, other reporters followed. Most sounded shocked. Few had read the *BMJ*. A grilling on local radio was followed by a roasting on national television.

On Saturday a tabloid carried my sinister picture—lip curled, eyes shifty—lifted from the Nine o'Clock News. Now I know why politicians appear with fixed smiles. BSkyB phoned to say a crew was on its way from Lincolnshire. The two young men—shell shocked after attempting to turn Skegness into interesting television—set up lights, read my article, and shot a sympathetic interview for Europe's hotel rooms.

A tough lady columnist phoned my wife, who disappointed her by supporting me. That evening, on a family outing to the theatre, my children pointed out news hoardings: YORKS DOC SPARKS CANCER STORM. At *The Rivals* I half expected Mrs Malaprop to lean over the footlights and ask me about mastoidectomy.

On Easter Sunday my father phoned, sounding as if he had had a hard time at church. Next morning I was beamed by satellite to Australia. The formula was becoming familiar—amiable technicians, terse producer, and lastly the presenter, charming until the microphones went live, then affecting outrage.

On Tuesday during a phone-in on local radio, an irate man said, "I just hope my sister isn't listening to this." It seemed to me he was speaking for everyone. Then, from a tiny studio, I was put through to Radio Oxford. After snatches of music on my headphones, I heard the interviewer speaking to an oncologist. For the first time in six days I heard a supportive voice on the air. I was close to tears.

Next day the handwritten envelopes started arriving, at first mainly from readers of a tabloid which had made me "Wally of the Week." Half the letters were abusive and hinted at castration: I replied with a fact sheet comparing testicular and breast cancer. The others were from women asking for mastectomy. The most upsetting was from a dying woman who wished I had written 10 years ago.

My own patients were unfazed. One grinned that before her hysterectomy she would write HANDS OFF on her chest. Another, worried about her family history, requested mastectomy after delivery.

A few weeks on, I can again start the day without a knot in my stomach. It was a surprise to find how paranoid one becomes under pressure. It was disappointing to find that the world's journalists still regard the breasts as sex objects. And it was interesting to hear how many women and doctors agree with me but won't say so for fear of the media.

COATS OF MANY COLOURS

My fourteenth graduation ceremonial, counting my own and other people's. Haven't missed one since becoming a consultant. The one annual chance for a professor to dress up in technicolor plumage and flaunt status. No opportunity for academic showmanship in NHS clinics—no framed diplomas on walls, like consulting rooms in cartoons. Pity. Might be fun to have clerk not only change names on the board but take down and put up framed degrees—all Latin, sealing wax, and *Iacobus Owen Drifus*. Give queue something to think about, what?

Each year resolve to arrive at graduation suave, cool, plenty of time, but medical faculty usually ends up dashing in, seconds to spare. Shouldn't squeeze in quick hysterectomy before the organ recital, but ceremonial seems like skiving, somehow. Frantic rush from operating theatre to great hall, then horrors, realise that gown hirers in different building. Accost nearest graduand—where did you get that gown? Graduand blinks, parents stare aghast—has university changed its mind after all? Eventually find Aladdin's cave of academic dress. Hand over ticket: man leafs laboriously through downmarket black gowns, ignoring hand signals that mine is red one at the end.

Edinburgh MD gown designed for draughty Scottish lecture hall in winter, not quarter mile sprint in July. Arrive glowing at hall, put on hat over perspiring forehead. Hat unbelievably silly, worse every year. Try different angles: look like either Statue of Liberty or Bart Simpson. Why no one tell me this before I apply for university? UCCA should organise show with catwalk, or at least send candidates illustrations of robes. Emeritus professor appears in elegant gown with sumptuous colours; under envious questioning admits it was run up to his own specifications by friendly tailor. Prettiest hat is Leeds PhD—broad brim, floppy top, like Queen Mum at Garter ceremony.

Line up in twos, introduce ourselves, worry whether gowns clash. Start walking—out of step, sign of academic integrity. Hood, attached by loop to shirt button, threatens to pull shirt up, strangle wearer. Parents turn heads slightly as we process down centre aisle. Column splits: up on to platform, turn and face congregation. Gosh, say parents, Bart Simpson asphyxiating. Sit down, adjust shirt, remove hat at last thank goodness.

Always enjoy ceremony, though know chancellor's speech by heart now. Watch graduands' faces: by turns blasé, embarrassed, amused, then anticipation and, at moment of truth, pure pleasure. Parents proud but more circumspect. Everyone self conscious— even chancellor on best behaviour, knows one hiccup would destroy magic. My delight tempered by realisation that I now identify with grey haired parents, not tanned graduands.

Afterwards sherry, strawberries, cameras. Congratulate pretty graduate. Pretty graduate reminds me we last met in pass-fail viva. Now my turn to be lost for snappy answer, but it doesn't matter. All smiles today: shared happiness of great life event. Birth of new doctors after long gestation. Or rather, christening: stress of labour gone but not forgotten. Only at this ceremony men too wear silly hats.

RAGS TO RICHES

In his monologue on menstruation, the comedian Ben Elton asks his audience what it would be like if men had periods. He imagines W G Grace speaking at a cricketing dinner. "There I was," he roars, "halfway to the wicket and what d'you you think— MY PERIOD STARTED!" His point is that if menses were masculine they would not be taboo.

After 20 years of talking to women about their periods, I should hate to menstruate. The human ovarian cycle is one of Nature's more heartless practical jokes. Sheep come into season once a year; rabbits are induced ovulators, but only women (and a few monkeys) have to cope with monthly incontinence of blood. I would resent carrying a handbag, queuing for inadequate toilets, and smiling through my uterine contractions.

Because I'm male I don't menstruate, and the same applies to most MPs and civil servants. This is why the government thinks it is reasonable to tax the menstrual flow. As if 37 years of monthly bleeds were not misery enough, HM Customs and Excise charge value added tax (VAT) on sanitary protection.

How much profit does the state make from menstruation? A packet of 40 sanitary towels costs £3 to £5 depending on the brand. A woman who uses a whole packet each month will spend £40 to £65 a year. With over 13 million menstruating women in Britain, the market could be worth £500 million a year, but the manufacturers of tampons give a more conservative estimate of £179 million—VAT on this figure amounts to over £30 million a year.

On current prices the average woman will pay about £100 tax on her periods during her life. A woman who consults you with genuine menorrhagia, however, will pay considerably more. A packet of 20 regular tampons costs about £1.74 but a packet of 40 super absorbent tampons costs £3.49. If you take a detailed history of menorrhagia you will find that some women pad themselves up with a tampon and more than one towel in order to go to work. Even if your patient ends up with a hysterectomy the state will still have made a profit from her disorder.

Services that are exempt from VAT include those of doctors, dentists, and opticians, and—perhaps less predictably—betting and gaming and the provision of credit. Zero rated items include the dispensing of prescriptions, aids for handicapped people, food, books, newspapers, houseboats, and children's clothes. The list gives an endearing insight into what the well educated British male considers important. Condoms, needless to say, are taxed at the full rate. AIDS, which has made condoms respectable, might change this, but can anything stop civil servants sniggering about sanitary towels?

Women don't complain because it isn't done to make a fuss about your periods. Women who reach positions of influence don't want to lose face by talking about menstruation, and in any case such women are usually comfortably off and postmenopausal. The sums are trivial—£30 million doesn't buy much nowadays—but the principle isn't. It is disgraceful to tax menorrhagia.

I-SPY HOSPITAL ARCHITECTURE

Visiting hospitals can be tedious. Whether you're an SHO seeking the personnel department or a professor searching for the postgraduate centre, you end up in a cul de sac by the boilerhouse or at an empty desk marked "Enquiries," wishing you were elsewhere. Next time, brighten your visit by spotting how a hospital's architecture reveals its history.

In a Victorian hospital, I-spy *portakabins*. Old buildings with sturdy joists and lots of space between wards are ideal for perching plasterboard sheds on roofs and flower beds. If you can't see them, follow signs marked "Academic Department of. . . ."

The 1930s were the golden age of hospital carpentry, with solid parquet floors, and I-spy *doors with handles* that actually work. These are quite unlike contemporary handles, which last about four weeks before falling off in a shower of small screws and powdered plywood.

The 1940s' contribution to hospital architecture was the Nissen hut—or, as it was later called, the doctors' residence. These buildings, originally dubbed "temporary" to fool the enemy, are marvellously durable. I-spy *wallpaper*, a tribute to the taste of wartime interior decorators who chose patterns of such timeless beauty that nobody can bear to replace them.

The fashion in the 1960s was to construct hospitals out of materials that had fallen off the backs of lorries. I-spy the *bottom half of a lift*, stuck between two floors with muffled sounds of engineers working above. Sixties' plumbing is easily recognised by its characteristic sounds: when someone somewhere empties a bath, every sink in the building gurgles. I-spy the *doctor* standing in front of such a sink. The basin behind him gloops and glugs, the patient stares wide eyed at his waistcoat, and the doctor gravely remarks, "No more curried eggs for me."

The 1970s saw the introduction of standardisation. Every British hospital was issued with an extremely large chimney. You rarely see smoke issuing from it: its purpose is to allow the hospital to be identified from the other side of town, so that visitors can navigate through the 1970s one way system. I-spy also *standard signposts*. NHS policy is to fill each post with as many signs as possible, in identical lettering and with randomised arrows, but always to omit the personnel department and the postgraduate centre.

In the 1980s architects decided to hide all hospital stairs. This was to symbolise a complete break from the previous century, when hospitals consisted mainly of staircases—the internal ones magnificent, the external ones functional. In a modern hospital, I-spy (eventually) the *concealed staircase*—cramped, unmarked, and reached through a door with no handles.

Progress in the nineties means shopping malls. The foyer of a British hospital now resembles a high street, with banks, newsagents, bookshops, and I-spy the *twee hairdresser*, "Doctor

53

McCurls." As patients move from hospital to community, shops are moving in the opposite direction. Soon all patients will be outside, the ground floor will be devoted to retailing, and the doctors will be undisturbed, up the hidden stairs.

A DOCTOR WRITHES

"**D**o you have any rules about entry?" I bellowed. This was the first time I had been to a nightclub in Yorkshire.

The man behind the half door leaned forward, grinned, and yelled, "Gotta be smartly dressed."

We agreed that in my black pinstripe suit, waistcoat, watch chain, and college tie, I was well on the safe side of the "no jeans" regulations. I paid £2.50 and entered. The music pounded even more loudly, lights flashed, and a mass of bodies seethed on the dance floor. Behind a railing on a mezzanine were more swaying people. There was a bar but hardly anyone stood beside it. Stroboscopes came on for a few seconds and went off. Multiple spotlights changed colour. It was like one of those 2 am television shows from Preston or Coventry, except that no one came up to me and started pulling faces.

When my students had invited me to join their celebrations I had envisaged discos I remembered from the sixties—people grouped by gender for most of the evening, shouted conversations, and intermittent dancing to records that jumped if you stamped your foot. The nineties version was a revelation: if you wanted to dance, you danced, and the club had a system of stimuli that plugged directly into your hypothalamus. Conversation was impossible. People joined the throng in groups, jumped around, and went away again. This was tribal, as far from the valse veleta as you could imagine, and in its way more sophisticated.

I could recognise nobody and began to think that my students, flushed with their exam success, had gone home. Then I saw them in the middle of the floor, where the music was loud enough to feel.

The beat thudded down from the roof and throbbed up through the floor. "Great sound system," yelled one, "pain threshold but no distortion." My body responded with Jacksonian movements— Hughlings Jackson, unfortunately, not Michael. One toe began to twitch, then a leg, then the other limbs joined in.

This was a purely physical experience—like swimming, except that one was immersed in sound rather than water. The enveloping rhythms made the ambience even more intrauterine, and like fetuses' our movements were only partially coordinated. I began to enjoy myself and writhed with growing gusto, though I drew the line at jumping up and down on the spot. Bald head nodding, paunch wobbling, I gyrated around my tiny personal space. The students pretended not to notice.

The onset of chest pain reminded me it was time to make an excuse and leave. In this freestyle place, however, no excuses were necessary and indeed it was difficult to catch the eye of one's pogo-sticking host. I drove sweatily home with my ears ringing. The first time I had experienced tinnitus was in 1965 after a Rolling Stones concert in a Cardiff cinema, where the deafening noise had come mainly from the screaming audience. I decided I could afford to sacrifice a few ear cells every quarter century.

TOWERING INFERNO

The hospital fire alarm is a litmus test. When it sounds, staff divide into two groups—those who quit the building and those who stay. The quitters are people for whom an emergency evacuation is welcome excitement to punctuate their day. The stayers think themselves so important that they must remain at their posts until flames lick their stethoscopes. Which group is right?

In 21 years of hospital life I have found a perfect negative correlation between fire alarms and fires. I've survived two hospital fires. In the first I was having tea in sister's office at night when

we heard feet scurrying in the ward above. We finished our tea and
went to investigate. I met a fireman dashing upstairs unrolling a
hose. After thoroughly dousing the male surgical patients' sitting
room he left.

A year later, I was in the same office when the same scurrying
began. Now an experienced registrar, I explained to the nurses that
the noise meant the hospital was on fire. This fire crew was even
more impressive: an officer dashed upstairs to the sitting room,
emerged with a smouldering television in his arms and ran outside,
where three fire tenders turned their hoses on it. It sat, black and
wet, in the car park for the rest of the week.

In those days the fire alarms didn't work. Since then the nation's
hospitals have been equipped with sophisticated devices that burst
into ear splitting life every time a man with a drill puts up a shelf
somewhere in the building. Doors close automatically, men with
bunches of keys and portable telephones march around and tell
you to stop working, enormous numbers of staff whom no one
has ever seen before congregate on the pavement, and fire engines
waa-waa their way to the wrong entrance.

Heroes in yellow helmets comb the hospital, find the man with
the drill, and tell him to stop. An older officer with a white helmet
searches the building again slowly, just to make sure it isn't on fire,
before allowing the men with the keys to turn off the alarms and let
people back inside.

This performance is repeated irregularly throughout the year
and rehearsals are held every week. Testing occurs in the middle of
a weekday morning, and is timed to coincide with the most short
tempered consultant's outpatient clinic. During that morning,
each sensor in the hospital is individually tested by someone who
walks around very slowly, setting off the entire system of bells and
hooters at unpredictable intervals.

In contrast to the false alarms, testing is associated with a
towering inferno. Smoke issues from the consultant's ears as he
tries to empathise amid the decibels. The patient, to whom
everything in hospital is strange, seems not to notice the nearby
klaxon, but becomes a little agitated as her doctor spontaneously
combusts while phoning the general manager. There should be a
notice: "If the alarm sounds, throw a bucket of water over the
nearest consultant."

George Dunea

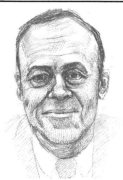

PERFUME

A pig lives in an apartment on the street next to ours, in the heart of downtown Chicago. Vietnamese by birth, it weighs 150 lb (68 kg), and its pot belly almost trails on the ground. Its adoring owners keep it as a pet, causing the neighbours to complain to the police. But the judge said that there was nothing in the condominium rules against pigs living in the building. Its immigration papers were in order, the green card obtained legally and not through a bogus marriage.

Why should the neighbours object so much? Are they afraid of bumping into their new neighbour in the elevator or at the laundromat? Do they think he will bring down property prices and put off Japanese investors? But the pig is polite, house trained, practically noiseless and odourless.

Yet people could understandably be revulsed by the thought of a pig next door in a society that has banished all smells from man or beast. For here the deodorant reigns supreme, in creams and sprays and roll-on bottles. Aluminium is still the main ingredient, but worry over Alzheimer's disease has spawned an interest in more "natural" deodorants. One highly recommended brand contains aloes, coriander, non-alcoholic witch hazel, vera gel, camomile tea, and xantham gum—the latter reassuringly described as vegetable.

Americans may not be alone in their aversion to odours. Some Buddhists find smells so repugnant that they spend days purifying themselves with incense. In the Book of Esther the young virgins shortlisted to replace Queen Vashti underwent 12 months' purification, six months with oil of myrrh, six with sweet odours, but

57

none with deodorants. Some human smells, however, function as pheromones: "I am coming home," wrote Napoleon to Josephine, "don't wash."

There must be millions of substances, each with it own characteristic smell, all of potential diagnostic value. Fetor hepaticus is well known, as is the fishy smell of non-specific vaginitis; also the uraemic breath, probably caused by amines formed in the gut by decomposing bacteria. In former days old nurses were said to be able to diagnose typhoid fever by the smell. Scientists have tried to characterise some of these substances by chromatography, but often ended up merely with pages of unidentifiable squiggles.

In the future better methods of on-line separation and characterisation may expand our diagnostic capabilities. Meanwhile imagination has anticipated science in the fictitious Grenouille, hero of Patrick Süskind's *Perfume*. This odd creature had an extraordinary sense of smell and could recognise people or identify the ingredients of even the most complicated perfume by merely sniffing them. To him even milk was quite different each day, depending on how warm it was, what cow it had come from, or what the cow had eaten. Every girl smelled differently and they overwhelmed him with such a plethora of odours that he would fall violently in love and then strangle them to forever possess the precious scent.

Imagine a physician, endowed with such a gift, walking around a ward and diagnosing by smelling all kinds of diseases, some old, some not yet even described. He would need no autoanalysers, not even routine blood tests. But he would also find it intolerable to have a pig next door.

BURNING DOWN
THEIR HOUSES

How thin is the veneer of civilisation. Remember how quickly it came off in Luis Buñuel's film of the elegant partygoers trapped by an invisible angel in a closed room. This time round the *Exterminating Angel*, the pathogen, is the AIDS virus and the vectors are said to be the very people who each day may be risking their lives treating the victims of the disease. Recently a senator wanted to send HIV positive doctors to prison. Will he also, as in the days of the plague, burn down their houses?

All this hysteria began when five people became HIV positive after being treated by a dentist who either infected them with his own blood or transmitted the virus from one patient to another. In a highly publicised case one woman subsequently developed clinical AIDS and the national newspapers displayed pictures of her wasted frame, describing how she had become emaciated, lost her hair, was covered with blisters and acne, and developed vomiting, cramps, diarrhoea, and unremitting fevers. Outrage and panic ensued, giving rise to widespread demands for compulsory testing of health workers.

By June Vice President Quayle had joined in the fray by announcing that mandatory testing was a good idea. The American Medical and Dental Associations at first opposed compulsory testing but later advised infected doctors not to do invasive procedures and to disclose their condition to their patients. Several states passed laws requiring hospitals to notify patients that they may have been exposed to AIDS through certain procedures. Finally, a senator introduced a bill in Congress imposing a $20 000 fine and a 10 year prison sentence for doctors who knowing they are infected carry out invasive procedures without telling their patients.

Yet so far a minuscule number of patients are believed to have been infected by health care workers. Some 6000 health workers in the United States (including 300 surgeons and 1200 dentists), are said to carry the HIV virus, and according to a mathematical model their chances of infecting a patient are exceedingly small. They pale into insignificance, a recent editorial suggested, compared with the enormous risks of smoking and car accidents that society is willing to tolerate.

But why limit testing to doctors and dentists? ask some. Why not to manicurists, hairdressers, or barmen? Why not test every patient? "Disgustingly," writes a surgical house officer, "if I contract AIDS from a patient I am told to stop performing surgery. No thanks," he goes on; "either I operate on all patients, regardless of my HIV status, or patients and surgeons should both have the option of selecting each other." He points out that some day his family responsibilities may take precedence over medicine.

Others have also alluded to the possible consequences of foolish legislation. What if those currently treating patients with AIDS were to question the wisdom of taking risks? Already inner city hospitals, where most of the AIDS victims are being treated, are experiencing shortages. Why be a hero, they might wonder, in a society that would show little sympathy if they themselves were to become infected in the course of carrying out their duties.

SURROGATES

It is by now generally established that people in possession of their wits have the right to refuse any treatment offered to them by their medical attendants. But what about patients who cannot make rational decisions because they are unconscious or mentally incompetent or likely to become so? Here the use of living wills and surrogate decisions, recently legitimised by new laws, may help doctors navigate across a perilous quagmire where ethicists and contingency lawyers lurk at every turn.

Since last December a new federal law requires hospitals and nursing homes to inform patients in writing of their rights to make health care decisions. They must document in the medical record that the patient was asked if he or she had made a living will or issued advance directives; they must also have established written policies on these issues; and they must inform and educate the staff about these policies.

While imposing an extra load of paperwork, these provisions should allow the public airing of issues often left unspoken. It is expected that the admission clerks will do the preliminary work. The doctor, starting off by knowing where the patient stands by merely looking at the bedside chart, should then feel more comfortable in opening a dialogue, discussing options, answering questions, and offering counselling.

For patients whose wishes were not spelt out in advance, a new law in Illinois gives doctors the power to appoint surrogates to make decisions on their patients' behalf. This applies only to terminal illnesses where death is imminent, to permanent unconsciousness, or to an irreversible state for which further treatment provides only minimal benefit. The doctor must first establish the presence of one of these conditions and have these findings confirmed by a second doctor. The law does not apply to incurable dementia or Alzheimer's disease.

To prevent abuse and as a safeguard in case the patient does indeed understand what is being done, the attending doctor must also ask patients if they agree to having a surrogate represent them. The doctor may then appoint one according to a spelled out hierarchy: guardian, spouse, children, parents, siblings, grandchildren, or a close friend. The surrogate may then act without a court order and can stop treatments such as ventilation, surgery, dialysis, blood transfusion, administration of drugs, and artificial feeding or hydration. In making decisions the doctor must henceforth regard the surrogate as though he or she were the patient. The law protects the doctor and the surrogate for decisions made in good faith, though not against "negligence" in carrying out their duties.

These two laws should help doctors in an area clouded by much uncertainty. But while confirming the primacy of the patient's wishes, they offer little help when relatives insist that futile treatments be continued. Although strictly speaking doctors cannot be forced to prescribe such treatments against their best judgment (such as indefinite ventilation or dialysis for a permanently comatose patient), fears of prosecution or malpractice suits generally result in such procedures being continued, often at a cost of millions of dollars.

Faced with escalating costs, hospitals have lately resorted to the courts, asking for permission to discontinue certain treatments such as ventilators. But the results have been mixed, and additional legislation may be needed to clarify these murky issues. As an ethicist put it recently, "the idea that patients have a right to demand any treatment in a system where 35 million people cannot even get a prescription is preposterous."

GEORGE DUNEA

CLOSING THE HOSPITALS

In many respects closing a hospital is tantamount to wiping out an entire community. It scatters people who have worked together for many years and who may never meet again. The nurses, always in high demand, are the first ones to move on, often at the first rumour of closure and even some time before the final word is out. Never again will nurse X call from intensive care at 2 am to tell you that Mr Jones in bed 2 has just vomited a pint of coffee grounds and that his vital signs are unstable. Then the doctors start admitting their patients to other hospitals and eventually stop coming. Later they may meet again at medical society functions; but lost for ever is the unique chemistry of a doctors' lounge where colleagues drank coffee and chatted about patients and many other things. Gone likewise will be the other workers, the librarians, the clerks, the guards; and there will be no more Christmas parties. Gone also is the silent majority, the patients, the other members of the family, some of whom had actually been born there. They too must now go to different hospitals, often to different doctors.

So far, 15 hospitals have closed in the Chicago area and several more are expected to follow suit. Located in the inner city and serving mostly the poor, they could not survive the present reimbursement policies and at last ran out of money. Even the survivors face an uncertain future, too strapped for funds to make improvements or replace obsolete equipment. They too may eventually close, perhaps because somewhere some higher power has decided that larger hospitals are more efficient or possibly more easily policed.

Chicago and London have the doubtful distinction of being sister cities in this respect; so that the Metropolitan Hospital where I worked some 30 years ago has also been closed. There it was, in the east end of London, small though not necessarily beautiful, but friendly, where people all knew one another. It had two medical wards, one for men and one for women. Everything was within easy reach; and it did not take 30 minutes and two elevator rides to get from one ward to another.

The hospital had five visiting attending physicians, each of whom made rounds on different days. There was a busy casualty

62

department, a daily outpatients clinic, and also a considerable tradition. Parkes Weber was said to have visited there and observed many of the rare syndromes he described in his book, some of which still hear his name. There were so many tabetics at outpatients that it sufficed for diagnosis to look at their pupils, test the ankle jerks and deep pain sensation, and stand them up for a Romberg's test. Curiosities included a large family with coexisting polycystic kidney disease and peroneal muscular atophy. Two Turkish sisters unaccountably both had carpal tunnel syndrome; and several Iranian nurses perpetually complained of lower abdominal pain. In the summer there was an outbreak of rubella with arthritis of the small joints of the hand and carpal tunnel syndrome, an entity that apparently had not yet been widely recognised at the time.

Now all that is gone. Yet could it be that these closures are a big mistake? Are little hospitals really that inefficient? Are these large monsters with their high costs, bloated bureaucracies, and a post office atmosphere truly more cost effective? It is not perhaps a grave evil and a disturbance of the right order of things, as Professor E F Schumacher once suggested, to assign to greater organisations functions that a smaller entity can do just as well?

SILICONE CASH COW

The use of silicone for breast augmentation began with Japanese prostitutes trying to suit the tastes of American soldiers and later grew into a vast American industry, a cash cow as some would have it. Until lately 150 000 women had silicone implants each year, for cosmetic reasons (80%) or for cancer. Then the Food and Drug Administration became alarmed by reports of untoward reactions such as capsular contracture, rupture, and autoimmune or scleroderma-like illnesses; and in November it called for a "voluntary" 45 day moratorium, saying it could not guarantee the long term safety of these implants.

In the maelstrom of diverse pronouncements that followed the *feminists* wanted women to have a choice but regretted their need for a certain stereotype of beauty that left them "implanted and ignorant," "gleefully misled for profit." *Consumerists* noted that cosmetic surgery was the most rapidly growing specialty, "whose experimental subjects were 78% female" and deplored the full page advertisements of a famous model selling breasts. They also blasted the profit hungry companies, even though the largest group of shareholders were pension funds.

Cancer support groups said their studies showed that 85% of recipients were satisfied, 90% of people believed silicone implants should remain an option, and 87% of mastectomy patients attributed their emotional recovery to having implants. Many *patients* also protested against the ban, saying that saline devices, the alternative, were far less aesthetically pleasing; but patients with complications sued or gave exhaustive interviews to the newspapers. The *plastic surgeons* were "surprised, upset, frustrated, flooded with calls." Pointing out that no device could ever be 100% safe, they none the less agreed that women should be fully informed of the risks of the procedure.

The *contingency lawyers* smelt blood and were seen circling. Some invested heavily in the business, buying $750 how-to-sue kits from advocacy groups, consolidating single cases into class action suits, confident that the women make credible witnesses and sympathetic victims. Several *columnists* thought the lawyers were destroying America's competitiveness and spirit of innovation, there being more lawyers in one single skyscraper than in the whole of Japan. The *free marketeers* thought that government agencies should stay out of people's business because they botch up everything they touch; also that their "experts" were biased and in conflict of interest, being paid $350 hourly for giving evidence. But the *newspapers* had a field day, hardly a week passing without sensational headlines and startling revelations.

And so the debate continued until April, when the Food and Drug Administration ruled from up high. It would allow implants only as part of strictly controlled clinical studies, with protocols, certifications, consent forms, data collection, and field inspectors to check compliance. They would be available to patients with cancer and to some 2000 women yearly for breast augmentation. "It's all over for silicone breast implants," said a prominent consumer advocate; but others predicted that women would soon be flocking south of the border as the cash cow relocates to greener pastures in Mexico and the Caribbean.

AT NIGHT

You live in a fine house with elegant children and obedient furniture when suddenly, in the first sweet sleep of night, you develop severe pain, perhaps accompanied by calor, rubor, tumor, and angor. How will you cope with this predicament under various circumstances in various parts of the world?

(1) If you should happen to be the emperor of China, a high ranking samurai, or the president of a multinational corporation, you may reasonably expect a sleepy doctor to arrive with his black bag to assuage your symptoms.

(2) If the above fortunate circumstances do not apply but the house call has not yet become extinct in your part of the world, a general practitioner may still come to see you. He may have a hard time examining you in a bad light in the middle of a sagging bed, but may nevertheless be astute enough to diagnose your leaking ulcer or classical panic attack.

(3) Working your way down the algorithm, you may possibly have an influential friend or relative who knows a doctor willing to come in the middle of the night, even if merely to determine that your dolor and angor are greatly exaggerated.

(4) You have neither friend nor relative nor influence. But you know of an agency that sends itinerant young doctors to take care of nocturnal true or pseudo emergencies.

(5) You could not get a doctor, young or old, to come to your house for all the gold in China, let alone in Japan; but a general practitioner will meet you at his surgery and at least examine you in a decent light and not in a king size bed.

(6) You could not get a doctor even if the entire Tokyo stock market crashed, but you can try your luck on the phone.

(7) You're on the verge of success. Unfortunately, the chap on the other end of the line does not seem to care even if you were the emperor's eldest son.

65

(8) The phone is "manned" by a formidable nurse practitioner whose job is to weed out the worried well—thereby increasing your angor and activating considerable furor.

(9) There is nobody to answer the phone; or your phone was disconnected because you did not pay last month's bill. So you get in the car and drive to the nearest emergency room.

(10) You don't have a car; it will not start; or it was repossessed for non-payment of due instalments. Your neighbour is in the same boat (with his car). You decide to take a midnight walk (in some neighbourhoods your last). Or call an ambulance that will charge more than it would cost to fix up both cars and possibly the boat as well.

(11) You are met by a stony faced clerk who wouldn't care if you were the dowager empress herself. You wait for hours to see the intern, a heavy sleeper. He orders every test under the rising sun, takes four views of your tumor, and sticks a needle in your rubor. He asks why you did not call your personal physician in the first place. He then phones his attending physician, who is at a poker game and of course does not know you from Adam's mother in law. You may be admitted to the hospital, a process that may be completed by sunrise, or you may be told to see your own doctor but come back if you don't get better.

(12) The meta-analysis is completed. Statistics indicate with a high degree of confidence that you should avoid getting sick outside regular business hours. You may safely read Shelley but do not arise from dreams in the first sweet sleep of night.

CLOUDS IN INTENSIVE CARE

The patient presumably lay somewhere under the tangled web of wires, his bed surrounded by the respirator, the auscultator, the carburator, the pulverator, the integrator, and the cardiogrump, all pulsing in unison. There would have been no way to listen with a stethoscope, not even if one could have been found on the unit.

It wasn't necessary, however. For two months the integrator had skilfully coordinated the movement of the various machines. All was calm as the nurse, exhausted after a gruelling three hour shift, was eating her sushi from a recyclable paper plate.

In a corner the ethics committee was still debating. It had been in session for three weeks after its latest reconstitution. Everybody had at last agreed that proper representation from the community should include a vegetarian priest, a fundamentalist muezzin, a presocratic engineer, a medicine man from Gambia, two officials from the shepherds' union, and a third year Hispanic schoolgirl. A torn copy of *Das Kapital* on the floor remained as sole evidence of the violent ethical polemic that had finally been settled in an uneasy compromise. All was harmony now, the muezzin chanting softly, the schoolgirl practising her multiplication tables. Quietly the nurse tiptoed into the room to borrow a screwdriver from the engineer to disconnect the cardiogrump. "It's OK," she said, "the machine has given its informed consent." Everybody looked relieved.

A little further on, the intensivity professor was lecturing to the residents. "It had started as focal cerebellar pediculosis," he explained, printing the words on the blackboard, the residents dutifully taking notes. "The process had spread through the foramen magnum and along the spinal cord to the abdomen," he explained. They had had to suck out the infected spleen through the pulverator, with immediate improvement in all haemodynamic parameters. Now the urology resident came in to ask something about a catheter. "It's not my patient," cried all the residents in unison. "It belongs to Smothers," explained a brain dead honours student, "and he is away taking a cardiogrump computerisation course." The patient's chart was nowhere to be found, until the urologist discovered that the chairman of the ethics committee was sitting on it to relieve his ailing back.

Then the nurse attempted to disconnect the cardiogrump. The ethics committee stood by with bated breath. All went well until suddenly the nurse's sushi plate was sucked down into the pulverator. The members of the ethics committee turned pale. The nurse by now looked distinctly emaciated. A lively discussion ensued on the ethics of hyperalimenting her on the spot. By now the pulverator had digested the soy sauce and the integrator had recalibrated his orchestra of machines. Strange waves appeared on the ausculta-tor and nobody could tell if they came from the patient or the cardiogrump. The neurologist looked for guidance to the ethics committee but found them deeply enveloped in the fog produced by the pulverised sushi plate. The intensivity professor looked puzzled. "I wish I had a stethoscope," he thought. He turned to the nurse, now busily filling in her time sheet, to at least borrow the screwdriver. By now the sushi cloud had filled the whole room. The waves on the ausculator could no longer be seen. Somewhere under the cloud the medicine man was murmuring an incantation. The patient opened the door and entered the room. He had been on a pass for 24 hours but had promised he would return. He looked at the disorder in his room, tightened the cord of his silk dressing gown, dutifully signed consent form 223A, and phoned for a taxi to pick him up from in front of the intensive care unit.

TRACKING
MEDICAL DEVICES

Within a period of about 40 years creative pioneers, often working under difficult conditions, have saved countless lives by developing a whole host of artificial organs and implan-table devices. They built these devices however they could, often facing great obstacles. Their progress was slow; they had successes but even more disappointments; and although the profit motive did not rank high in their minds, they soon discovered that eventually industry had to become involved to effect the final transition from the workbench to the bedside. Their eventual success, it is fair to say, can be attributed to an environment that helped unleash the creative energy of a generation of such ingeni-ous investigators.

This creative energy is now sadly being stifled to death. Witness the Safe Medical Devices Act of 1990, passed by Congress with the laudable intent of protecting the consumer. Apparently enacted in response to problems with the generic drug industry, it requires a tightening of the manner in which the Food and Drug Administration (FDA) reviews new medical devices before approving them for marketing.

This new measure puts increased responsibility on manufacturers to demonstrate the safety and effectiveness of their products. Though passed in 1990, it has been implemented slowly because of staffing shortages at the agency and complaints from industry. But sometime in 1993, according to recently published regulations, the FDA will require manufacturers to track millions of pieces of foreign material implanted into human bodies. For each device the manufacturers will need to develop a system to keep track of the lot number, the batch number, the serial number, the date it was shipped, the name, address, phone number, social security number of the prescribing physician, the surgeon, the physician regularly following the patient, and the patient.

There are pages of additional "requirements and responsibilities," rules for distributors, requirements about notification if the devices are "explanted," if they are returned to the distributors, if the patient dies; and detailed records will need to be kept for the government inspectors. All vascular graft prostheses fall under these rules, as do heart valves, pacemakers, infusion pumps, nerve stimulators, and breast, tracheal, and testicular prostheses, though mercifully not tracheostomy tubes and peritoneal dialysis catheters.

The whole thing promises to be a nightmare—just keeping track of perhaps 50 000 dialysis patients with prosthetic vascular grafts, let alone some 10 million other devices, boggles the mind. Nor is it clear what the manufacturers will do with all this paper or the FDA with the information; most likely they will just file it away. Yet despite a storm of protests the agency seems determined to press on regardless. It will impose an enormous burden on manufacturers and distributors, on hospitals and physicians; and the cost will eventually be passed on to the patients and the taxpayers. That such a law should have been passed in the first place goes a long way to explaining why American industry has lost its competitive edge. It may account for the public's disenchantment with its politicians and its interest in an alternative to the two main presidential candidates.

Tony Smith

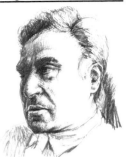

EXERCISE AND THE ENRAGED MOTORIST

I've stopped driving in London and become a pedestrian—and I now find motorists intolerable. In particular I am irritated by their use of their horns. Hardly ever is this legitimate—an audible warning of approach. Much more often they use the horn as a means of abusing other drivers. If a horn is sounded in central London it is usually a series of blasts carrying a message such as "Why are you driving so badly/slowly/close to me?" or "Wake up, the traffic lights have changed." Equally vexing to the pedestrian is the motorist who drives up outside a house or a block of flats and uses his horn instead of getting out of the car and using the doorbell. Sounding a horn in these circumstances shows arrogant indifference to the world outside the car; it is also illegal, since the horn should not be sounded if the vehicle is stationary, nor for that matter after dark.

The underlying cause of these inappropriate uses of the horn is, I believe, lack of exercise. The urban motorist is, almost by definition, someone who doesn't like walking or cycling and who prefers being in a warm, music filled car to being out on the street. Someone who takes no exercise never gets the adrenaline flowing in a normal way and certainly never experiences the pleasurable physical collapse at the end of a full day's hill walking or five sets of tennis, when the adrenals are presumably empty. Instead of taking exercise the urban motorist becomes angry; and there may well be some deeply natural biological mechanism whereby a body

71

deprived of physical causes for the sympathetic neurones and the adrenals to get to work finds psychological causes as a substitute.

Does the enraged horn-tooting motorist do much harm? He certainly does no good to his own cardiovascular system: hypertension, tachycardia, and arrythmias are all recognised responses in the excited driver. He also contributes to the frenzied hyperactivity of so many road users in Britain, competing with one another in a series of traffic light drag races. We really do need to find more and better ways of calming traffic by a combination of physical changes to roads and psychological changes in drivers.

In countries as far apart as Norway and Australia I have observed a different attitude to cars and driving. Cars are seen as boring machines for transportation, not expressions of the driver's virility and personality. Few people there buy GT or turbo models; when the lights change people move off slowly and non-competitively, and the horn is rarely used. There are other factors that contribute to this saner attitude to driving, including traffic police who really enforce speed limits, strict controls on drinking and driving, and courts which impose tough penalties. But I suspect that the main factor is that these are countries in which most motorists take plenty of physical exercise.

THIRD WORLD DEBT

One of the most heartening recent achievements in medicine has been the success of the World Health Organisation's campaign to make immunisation against the common fevers available to all children around the world. Nearly 80% of children are now being immunised, even in remote mountain and desert regions.

It makes little sense, however, to improve the health of the world's children if we are then going to starve them. Many African and Asian countries face economic problems all too familiar to mortgage debtors in Britain: they were lent money by eager bankers in the boom years of the '70s and '80s and now cannot afford to pay the interest, let alone repay the debts. We hear a lot about rescheduling and writing off Third World debts, but Africa's debt rose from $212 billion in 1986 to $272 billion in 1990, and there seems little chance that it will be reduced in the foreseeable future.

There are many reasons why Africa and much of Asia are so poverty stricken, some of them familiar—fortunes spent on armaments and rapidly rising populations. But one reason for the economic problems of the Third World stands out as being directly attributable to the rich Western countries. We pay them far too little for their exports.

Goodness knows they are trying to climb up the economic ladder. African countries have steadily improved their agricultural performance, increasing output by around 3% a year in the 1980s. The problem is that the West has been paying ever lower prices for the products that the Africans sell. In the past five years the volume of exports from Africa has risen by 7·5% while their unit value has fallen by 24 points. In other words, developing countries are working ever harder to grow more crops such as tropical fruits, sugar, coffee, tea, and cocoa and earning less for their efforts. These countries need export revenues to balance their trade and pay for vital imports such as medicines and machines. If their cash crops earn poorly their only answer is to increase production— often at the expense of food for their own people.

If the widening gap between the rich and the poor nations is an inevitable consequence of the operation of a free market system then we have to change the system. From time to time reports such as that of the Brandt commission appear, calling for steps to be taken to redress the economic imbalance between the northern and southern hemispheres. Nothing much seems to happen. Multinational companies talk about their duties to their shareholders— arguing that these absolve them from having any international social responsibilities. The coming years are going to see enormous upheavals in the world's economy as the countries of the former Soviet empire are put back on to their financial feet. We in the West should not lose patience with the poorer countries; we should use the peace dividend to give them more help.

TONY SMITH

BEING ILL IS HEALTHY

An elderly friend of mine has recently had a stroke and is now living in a nursing home, and it's a light, cheerful, pleasant place. But her grandchildren, who are in their 20s, are reluctant to visit her. They don't like institutions and they are uncomfortable in the company of someone who is obviously unwell. They are just not used to illness.

By the end of this century most young adults in Western countres will have passed through childhoods with no more serious illness than chickenpox and the occasional sore throat. Born in 1934, I had measles and mumps, yellow jaundice (hepatitis A), and appendicitis—and I was let off lightly. Measles meant two weeks in bed in a darkened room eating a light diet, but that was all. Being "ill in bed" had compensations, however, such as time to read and parental attention. Nevertheless, some of my friends at school had to endure months of forced bed rest for rheumatic fever; a couple had tuberculosis and had to go away to sanatoriums. No close friends died, but we knew of children who did. So we all grew up aware of illness, having been sick and having visited the sick. People had babies at home and died at home. We were aware of our mortality.

Nowadays with effective immunisations the greatest threat to child health is accidents. The same is true of the adult years; a substantial fraction of all people in countries such as Britain reach the age of 60 never having had any illness that kept them away from work for as long as a week. (It used to be said that civil servants were expected to take two weeks' sick leave a year on top of their holidays. Is that still true?)

The conquest of serious illness is so obviously an advance that it might seem odd to question it, but I wonder whether we are distancing ourselves too far from the realities that are part of human existence. Many children are not only never sick—they have never been seriously hungry or even cold. Recent surveys have shown that many have never experienced physical exhaustion. These are very basic feelings, and our responses to them are buried in our genes, waiting to be expressed. Perhaps we need to have at least some of these experiences in order to be able to cope later in life with personal illness, bereavement, and disasters. Of

74

course I am aware that emotional traumas remain all too common, with children experiencing the miseries of bullying, parental abuse, and the stresses of unemployment and poverty—and that these leave scars as deep as those of illness. But most children grow up in secure, happy homes and the question I am putting is whether we have removed too many of the natural stresses. Exercise is needed to strengthen the bones; is some experience of illness and stress needed as part of growing up?

TREES

Watching a tree grow requires patience and time, and in my 50s I find I have too little of both. Trees are the only familiar living structures that outlive man and planting them, nurturing them, and restoring their health gives a feeling of making history. I should like—now—to have planted more trees when younger, but this is the sort of wisdom that cannot easily be passed on to the next generation. Indeed giving parental advice to young adult children is mostly a waste of effort (though points may be scored for giving accurate, relevant facts when asked for them). Telling my children to plant trees while they are still young enough to watch their efforts grow to maturity is not only likely to be ineffectual it is also, in practical terms, pointless since none of them has a plot of land in which to do the planting.

It is the land or the uncertainty about it that makes the problems. The ideal tree planting setting is the family home in the country with enough land to be able to accept a few decent sized trees and a likelihood that the place will stay in the family for a few generations to come. These concepts are totally contrary to twentieth century man's concern with social and geographical mobility. I have left a few trees planted around houses sold long ago, and I envy those friends and acquaintances who can look at a substantial tree and claim it as their own. This is one advantage to living in the tropics: starting from scratch a garden can be filled with trees in as little as 20 years.

Here in Britain our most beautiful hardwood trees, the oaks and beeches, London planes, and imports such as cedars, need a full century to reach their majestic maturity, and planting them is an act of faith. But every tree planted is a contribution to the slowing of global warming and the improvement of the environment; carbon dioxide is fixed in wood. In 200 years when the trees are fully mature the problems of atmospheric pollution will either have proved overwhelming or will have been solved.

So, in a pale imitation of Johnny Appleseed, I shall continue to encourage people to plant seedling trees or saplings or even grow them from seed. This is not as frustrating as it sounds. Fast developers such as the catalpa or Indian bean and many evergreens, once established, will grow a metre a year in their adolescence. They do slow down later. And even without your own land it may still be worth while. All you really need is permission to plant in a location where you can watch the growth and there seems a reasonable probability that the young tree(s) will not be uprooted or felled in the next few years.

IS CANCER NATURAL?

Health educators in Western countries are—quite justifiably—pleased with their efforts to reduce the numbers of people dying of stroke and heart disease. Nevertheless, people have to die of something, and the declining mortality from heart disease is being matched by increases in deaths from cancer. Another factor in this changing pattern is the increase in the average age of the population; cancer is predominantly a disease of the elderly, doubling in incidence every 10 years after the age of 30, and the most very old people have malignant cells in some of their organs if these are examined carefully after death.

Yet for most people cancer is one of the big fears as they grow older. They fear cancer partly because they equate the disease with inevitable rapid death and partly because they believe that death from cancer is inevitably painful and distressing.

Doctors have a big public education job on their hands if, as I believe they should, they are to convince people that cancer is as natural a part of aging as wrinkling of the skin and greying of the hair. It occurs as frequently in aging domestic animals and pets as in their owners. The explanation of the dramatic increase in frequency of cancer with age has yet to be agreed by research scientists, but a decline in the efficiency of the immune system is one important factor.

What is needed is a substantial change in attitudes based on better understanding of the realities of cancer. The two central beliefs held by most people are, after all, wrong. Many cancers have a better prognosis than progressive neurological disorders such as motor neurone disease and than common conditions such as heart failure, emphysema, or cirrhosis of the liver (ignoring the effects of organ transplantation, which can be offered to only a few thousand people each year in Britain). And though dying of cancer may be painful and need specialist care for control of symptoms, in many cases it is not.

If I were given the opportunity to choose my way of death I would elect to die at the end of my natural lifespan, with my mind unaffected by disease, and I should like to have a few months between the recognition of my fatal illness and the actual moment of death. Such a set of requirements rules out dropping dead from heart disease, a ruptured aneurysm, or a stroke or progressive decline from dementia. Some of the common cancers do, however, offer a fair chance of filling the bill.

Of course we should press on with attempts to prevent cancer, but—as with heart disease—the main emphasis should surely be on preventing premature deaths. Death in old age is natural, and if we can be persuaded that cancer is part of that natural process then some of the fear it induces should be relieved.

SOCIAL MOBILITY UP AND DOWN

Even 40 years ago, when medical students and engineers were said to be less clever than students of classics and philosophy, all university students were in the top quartile of intelligence quotients. More recently competition for places in medical schools has made the profession an intellectual élite, and today doctors are right at the end of the distribution curve of intelligence.

In this era of health screening, indicators such as blood pressure and cholesterol are measured repeatedly and we have all learnt to recognise that lower readings on later measurements may simply be due to the phenomenon of regression to the mean. This concept also applies to the inheritance of characteristics such as height—very tall or very short parents tend to have children who are closer to the average.

Given, then, that doctors are substantially brighter than average, we should expect the phenomenon of regression to the mean to result in our children being—on average—less clever than we are (though some will be more clever, too). Indeed this is true of all families with parents who are university graduates. Yet this is an idea that makes many people feel uncomfortable—especially perhaps those who were themselves upwardly socially mobile.

Previous generations of the middle classes were able to look after their less bright children by sending them to exclusive schools to acquire social skills and confidence. With the right accent and the right social contacts middle class occupations could be found for them all. Not all that long ago medical schools and Oxbridge colleges made a virtue of offering places to the children of their former graduates—if a lad could play rugby football and make a bit of an effort he could always become a general practitioner. It is not only the metamorphosis of general practice into a demanding specialty that has changed this attitude of benevolent privilege; our competitive, meritocratic society now insists that entrance to higher education is based on examination results and not on parentage.

Sociologists calculate that around 10–15% of each generation of children born into social classes III, IV, and V make the transition upwards to the professions and managerial occupations. Less attention has been paid to the corresponding movement downwards, yet it certainly occurs. Other cultures seem to have accepted the reality of occupational mobility rather more easily than the British—probably because our educational and social systems are still so class ridden. In each generation some parents and children will need to face these realities, but they need not feel guilty or disappointed if they value each other as individuals. And because they are so far to the right end of the distribution curve, doctors will need to—and should—take a lead in this change in attitudes.

BEHIND THE SPEAKER

I go to fewer meetings nowadays and no longer have to report them; instead I can sit back, enjoy any talks that are enjoyable, and make my own unspoken criticisms of the contributions.

The best speakers seem to talk without obvious effort and without looking at their notes, making a few jokes and asides, obviously comfortable, assured, and getting pleasure from the occasion. Perhaps because these experienced lecturers make it seem so easy, young doctors speaking at a meeting for the first time often seem to think that it is indeed easy and that they can get up and give a spontaneous talk with no preparation beyond some scrappy notes.

A very few of us are natural performers who can speak on any topic with little forethought, improvising on our feet; but most of us are ordinary and fallible. Without preparation all too many speakers stumble on, losing their way in their handwritten notes, peering in a puzzled way at slides as if they'd never seen the data before, hardly ever finishing a sentence but starting another one instead. Their talks may include some factual information but it is commonly presented so badly as to be unintelligible; the presentations have no obvious structure and no clear conclusions and cast a suffocating cloud of boredom over the proceedings.

So how do the polished performers achieve their results? Part of the answer is that they have done it many times before, but by no means all experienced speakers are good at it. Talking to good lecturers who have become friends, reading scientific biographies, observing speakers in the hours before they speak—the evidence from these sources is clear and uniform: the good speakers have put in hours of work. They have recognised that a polished performance is just that: a stage presentation rehearsed as carefully as an actor's. Most top speakers have not only written a text but also rehearsed it, checking the timing to the last minute, running the slides through until they have become part of the script. Often they learn the talk by heart—just as actors do. (I'm always amazed at the ability of aging stage performers to learn vast parts such as Lear.)

Of course the best lectures are often set pieces that have been presented many times before, and like an actor performing Hamlet the lecturer becomes more assured after the first night; the mechanics become easier and attention can then be given to fine tuning, fitting the presentation to the audience.

Nevertheless, even if a young speaker knows that his talk will be a one off he will give a good performance only if he works at it. A 20 minute presentation may require a week's hard work, but it may also be a turning point in an academic career. The big differences between individuals, said Charles Darwin, are not in their abilities but in their willingness to work.

David Widgery

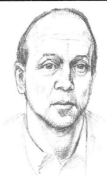

SICKNESS AND
THE NEW
UNEMPLOYED

Tower Hamlets was never really in on the roaring eighties, except in the rather dubious form of Canary Wharf, so it is now suffering from a double whammy of structural decline and recession. Those made unemployed in the long term by the closure of the docks and the river based industries have had virtually to give up hope of a job. Tragically, so have a lot of school leavers. According to age they drift variously towards chronic depression, psychosomatic illness, bitter despair, petty crime, dope of various sorts, and cathode tube addiction. All experience the progressive paralysis of will which chronic UB40ism generates.

But over the past year they have been joined by the new unemployed, skilled east end artisans from the building, engineering, and manufacturing sectors whom I have never previously known to be out of a job for more than a few weeks. Privatised, deregulated, and deunionised during the Thatcher clearances, they have had to travel further and work harder with no redress for bad conditions. But whether it was building Disneyland, burying cable television, or fitting the channel tunnel, there was always something. Now there's nought and they sit at home half heartedly fitting dado rails and cut price kitchen units, with the extended families who relied on their remittances unexpectedly broke. So too are luckless small businessmen of the enterprise culture, the redundant industrial workers who were pressured into taking out bank loans to get up their own companies, buy their vans, and set up as subcontractors. But now Enterprise Florists and Essex Piping are well and truly stuck in the economic gridlock which is east London. Not only has their work dried up but the cost of their borrowing has soared.

I now see many cases of "Small business sciatic syndrome," the rather exaggerated lumbago characteristic of a self employed central heating engineer who needs a two month sick note. Not because he'll be entitled to a bean from "the social," but if I sign the forms the banks will give him a moratorium on his repayments. Add to them retail workers whom cash flow makes let go, the service industry workers newly sacked by British Telecom and the city banks, and casualties of the casual catering trade and it's a very sizable blip. The optimists say, "I've not got a job like, but I'm still with an agency." The rest just look shifty when you ask for an occupation. The implications for medical workload are grim. We are familiar with prolonged unemployment's ill effects on health and know it is the single most potent generator of family poverty. But there is growing evidence that after a bumper year of NHS spending, post-election austerity and a public sector squeeze are likely. Medical business will boom, regrettably, on the basis of everyone else's recession.

FOOT SOLDIERS OF MENTAL ILLNESS

I suspect that the community psychiatric nurse is the most under appreciated member of the inner city primary health care team. District and practice nurses have a much longer professional history and a sharper identity. Health visitors have more career development and the undoubted kudos of dealing with the care of the under 5s. Everyone knows, or thinks they know, what the receptionists, midwives, practice managers, and physios do. And, for some reason that entirely escapes me, surveys continually show that the public adore their family doctors.

But the community psychiatric nurses, the foot soldiers of mental illness, are seriously undervalued. It is simply impossible for general practitioners to treat the torrent of emotional disturbance which comes into an inner city surgery, often in crisis, themselves. I have neither the time nor the skills—nor, these days, the therapeutic optimism. Medication is seldom the answer. And the hospital psychiatric service in east London, its beds and staff constantly shrinking while workload goes up, has its work cut out dealing with the acute and psychotic emergencies. So the community psychiatric nurses have filled the vacuum, training themselves and developing their specialty as they go along.

I say all this with a certain bitterness. For the past 12 months one of the community psychiatric nurses who does sessions at our health centre has been on prolonged sick leave and his replacements have been patchy and intermittent. The quality of care we can offer patients has undoubtedly deteriorated. We have documented cases of suicide attempts which should have been prevented; heroin users and problem drinkers who, untreated, have matured into preventable long term psychiatric morbidity. Predictably the remaining nurse is under immense pressure and the delay in getting community counselling is now nearly as long as the wait for a hospital outpatient appointment.

So last week we learnt with genuine delight that a permanent new community psychiatric nurse had been appointed. Then four days after the appointment we were informed, by phone, of a comprehensive cash freeze on the community budget (apparently to ease "overspending"—that is, underfunding—in the acute sector). All posts are frozen, no agency or pool staff will be available, all training has been cancelled, and no order forms above essential supplies will be signed. The new community psychiatric nurse is dehired, the (agency) caretaker who provides security for us and the evening receptionists go, and the bank health visitor also covering for sick leave goes back to the bank.

This is the reality of government assurances about trusts stopping end of financial year crisis. It is the sad truth behind the Royal London Hospital and Community Services Trust's promises to extend and improve its primary health care services. The salary bonuses, perks, and severance pay of the rapidly changing managers and executives who have achieved this cock-up are, of course, now confidential. But I can't help feeling they would be better spent on NHS staff who actually work with patients.

DAVID WIDGERY

DOCTORS AND MUSICIANS

The intricate interrelation of musicians, doctors, and ill health remains fascinating. Part of its interest lies in the chance it gives to appreciate the subjective experience of illness. Schumann suffered from severe and badly treated bipolar disease but wrote some of his most serene music during manic phases. Beethoven's late string quartets were written from the tonal prison of profound deafness while he endured the savage pain of pancreatitis, with both conditions inflecting the work's sonorities. Schubert's haunting late piano sonatas were composed at the time when he became aware that he was terminally ill with syphilis. Among jazz musicians Thelonious Monk may well have suffered from a schizophrenic type illness and certainly played knight's move piano but Bud Powell and Charles Mingus, whose bizarre behaviour was labelled mental illness, were more probably reacting to racial and physical abuse.

Ravel, who died after ill advised neurosurgical treatment, is not the only musical genius to be poorly served by the medical profession. Gershwin's death was from an astrocytoma which, according to the medical historian John O'Shea, might well have been operable if diagnosed more promptly. This seems to be an example of the general syndrome of medical indecision when confronted with eminent patients. Beethoven's otosclerosis was certainly compounded by treatments of the outer ear that caused a secondary iatrogenic otitis externa, and Paganinni is only one of many musicians whose syphilis was worsened by "therapeutic" mercury poisoning. Many of the geniuses of black America from Scott Joplin to Lester Young have received racist and incompetent medical attention. Not that musicians are always easy to treat—the physical strain of travel and performance and related fondness for tobacco and alcohol affecting classical heroes like Beethoven, Scriabin, and Liszt as much as jazz musicians.

These thoughts were prompted by the unexpected death of Miles Davis who, despite bouts of (self cured) heroin addiction, a hip fracture related to sickle cell disease, and maturity onset diabetes, was widely judged to be in the throes of a fourth renaissance. Certainly friends who saw him recently on the west coast now painting as well as composing ("Aria" was one of his

84

finest ever records) thought him better than the gaunt irritable despot I remember in the '70s, which his autobiography now reveals were times of addiction and ill health. In some ways Davis demonstrates in his music the impact of overcoming addiction. Although he had been a heroin-dependent bebop tiro, his classic quintets were achieved only after he had cleaned up. The ravishingly expressive music he went on to make, both in sickness and in health and quite comparable to that of Ravel or Schumann, can teach us about human indomitability, the surges, setbacks, and renaissances of creativity, and about emotional suffering and joy. And thus perhaps how to understand and treat our patients better.

THE PRINCE AND THE PSYCHIATRISTS

It is a pity that Prince Charles's oration to the 150th anniversary meeting of the Royal College of Psychiatrists in Brighton engendered so little comment. There was no repeat of the drubbing of Mies van der Rohe's Mansion House tower and Peter Ahrend's design for the National Gallery extension at the Royal Institute of British Architects in 1984 or of his more recent chiding of general practitioners for our lack of sympathy for alternative medicine. No psychiatric carbuncles or other gross sepsis were diagnosed by the prince, who was in self mocking deprecatory mode and radiating an asphyxiating niceness. It was, in fact, a standard issue royal speech, which could equally well have been about wild geese, the disabled, or Kalahari bushmen. He may need his head examined, he averred, but he thought that we doctors were all jolly good chaps for devoting ourselves to the relief of mental illness. And he was a jolly good chap for telling us that we were jolly good chaps.

In truth, it wasn't such a bad speech and when psychiatrists as well as the mentally ill usually get such a bad press—no, Prince Charles had not yet seen *Silence of the Lambs*—everything helps.

What worried me was not the attitude of the prince but that of the psychiatrists, who received him with an extravagant show of deference. The mood of the packed lecture hall was elated to the point of fatuity and the speech of welcome was downright grovelling. You would not have needed to be a republican (or a Finn or a physicist) to be puzzled by the sight of over 800 of the most experienced clinical practitioners of psychological medicine in the world listening, in near trance, to what they would have dismissed as bien pensant platitudes if they had been spoken by the chair of the league of friends. But the conference was intoxicated by the physical presence of the prince and his small retinue of Sussex mayors, lord lieutenants, chiefs of police, and so on. We were, as everyone kept telling us, so fortunate to have his presence.

The problem is not the prince but the professions, who nowadays seem to have convinced themselves that the only way to get back in touch with the voice of the common man is to invite the heir to the throne along. For this need for overt and symbolic royal patronage, so important nowadays to the leaderships of the royal colleges, is symptomatic of an inability or even fear of thinking for oneself and the future of one's profession. Indeed, it is still more disturbing in as far as it replaces the essentially republican spirit of scientific inquiry, for which psychiatrists in particular have had to fight so hard, with a quasi mystical sentiment which looks instead for regal intellectual guidance presumably in the knowledge that it will not be foreign or modern.

For what Charles promulgates is an implausible return to some wholesome, cosy, reintegrated world where all the nasty bits go away and instead of homelessness and closures and opt outs we can have long chats with the patients about Jung. The royal touch used to refer to the belief that when the monarch's fingers brushed against certain infections, usually smallpox, a magical charge flowed and promoted healing. Charles II used it extensively to consolidate the restoration of the monarchy and it has had a recent revival in the context of AIDS. But the seance at Brighton must be the first recorded case of the royal touch being applied not to the patients but the doctors.

AIDS FAREWELLS

The impact of AIDS on the artistic world is impossible to ignore. The night I saw the English National Opera's magnificent new production of Verdi's *Don Carlos*, Peter Jonas dedicated the performance to the memory of the composer, broadcaster, and critic Stephen Oliver and spoke movingly from the curtain of the beauty and honour of men's love for each other as expressed in the duet between Don Carlos and Rodrigo at the end of act one. In July, Maina Gielgud, director of the Australian Ballet, paid tribute from the same Coliseum stage to the dancer and ballet teacher Kelvin Coe, who had just died in Melbourne after a courageous battle against AIDS. The benefit performance of *Guys and Dolls* in memoriam of Ian Charleson was another superb and moving evening. The proximity of death in each case served to make the vitality of the performance still more ardent.

And who cannot be deeply moved by the bravery and defiance of Derek Jarman, who in the face of publicly acknowledged HIV disease has continued to make remarkable films and publish a diary that deserves to be a medical as well as a literary classic? Just before his death the American painter Keith Haring produced one of the most poignant images yet of this dreadful epidemic. It was a brilliant coloured acrylic pattern covering the top part of the painting in Haring's distinctive hieroglyphics which, as he abandoned painting through fatigue, loses its symmetries and disintegrates into falling ribbons of colour.

I don't wish to argue any privilege for death from AIDS. All premature death, regardless of diagnosis, must be mourned on an equal basis. But it seems to me that a grotesque act of denial is still going on in the public sphere about both the losses AIDS is inflicting on human society and the scale of the disease. Its particular characteristics—a retrovirus with long incubation period, sexual spread, vertical transmission, and eventually fatal outcome—make it particularly hard to come to terms with. Although the basic science of the disease has been elucidated with remarkable speed, the magnitude of the problem and the suffering it has already caused are taking far too long to sink in. It is gay people themselves who have done most to combat the disease and effectively spread ideas of safer sex. But when over 100 000 gay pride marchers, including many with HIV and AIDS, filled London's Brockwell Park to celebrate Europride Day, it was unmentioned by the same press that had been doing mental gymnastics trying to explain heterosexual spread in Birmingham. The unspoken attitude is still, "You've only yourselves to blame," although AIDS is no more a gay disease than German measles is German. It seems quite crazy that, although AIDS is second only to accidents as a cause of death among American men aged 25–44 and the sixth commonest cause of death among women of that age group, the subject remains taboo in the US presidential campaign.

There is a still more sinister overtone to the continuing non-coverage of the scale of the disease in Africa, another unspoken curse, as if it is now time to pull up the ladder from a continent we no longer need to exploit and never much liked. I sometimes just long for someone in power to acknowledge the scale of the loss and to offer to lend a hand. And mean it, not just say it.

THE ZOO TOO

Those still infatuated with the "free market" no doubt see marked similarities between London Zoo and the London teaching hospitals. They have in common high costs, distinguished architecture, nineteenth century ambitions, and too few late twentieth century paying customers. One might, unkindly, add that the traditional teaching hospital consultant had an attitude to NHS patients not entirely dissimilar to that of a Regent's Park spectator to the animals. But it is symptomatic of the process of decivilisation now rampant that we are even considering the closure of London Zoo, which remains, scandalously, the only national zoo in the world that gets no direct financial support from central or local government. And it is still more worrying that the great London teaching hospitals are being forced to announce, on an almost weekly basis, unplanned and destructive cuts in staff and clinical services.

Major metropolitan centres whose pursuit of scientific excellence as well as popular wellbeing has benefited the nation for over a century are being cynically driven into bankruptcy by a government which has abnegated its civic responsibilities to the capital.

The zoo has an outstanding record in anatomy and veterinary science and, far from being anti-animal, has a world reputation for breeding endangered species in captivity. Its architecture, from Decimus Burton's original layout, through Belcher's heroic Mappin Terraces, Lubetkin's Chaplinesque penguin pool, and Hugh Casson's elegant elephant house, to Lord Snowdon's remarkably durable aviary, is brilliantly juxtaposed. For generations of young city dwellers it has been the introduction not just to zoology but to biology, ecology, and the diversity of species. And, if anything, it is an underused tonic for grownups, who might find it better for depression than amitriptyline.

As for the London teaching hospitals, their contribution to science, research, and specialist and general medical education is immense and something from which we all profit. Inevitably the costs of sustaining this work as well as the high demands of Londoners and those often ill people who still flock to the capital would make their services "expensive." Yet many of us who provide services in community and primary care or lead hospital services outside the capital were often inspired to do so because of the teaching we received in London. Contrary to the implication of the recent King's Fund report, I have yet to find a single GP who believes that further teaching hospital closures are going to help primary care. What is happening is the triumph of accountancy over science. And the robbing of a broke Peter to pay a penurious Paul.

Butchering giraffes and converting teaching hospitals to luxury hotels deserve to become symbols of laissez-faire gone mad as much as selling off cemeteries. These acts of desecration are made all the more shocking by the news that, while we can no longer afford the capital's zoo or teaching hospitals, the government is intent on carrying on regardless with the European fighter bomber costing over £22 billion, a macabre fantasy which now lacks any military virtue it might once have possessed. As the Victorian music hall artiste The Great Vance used to sing, "Walking in the Zoo/Is a better thing to do." Especially as I calculate that by cancelling this ariel farrago we could afford to write off all current debts and fund the zoo and the hospitals properly and still have enough left for 500 000 council houses and 20 years' food for some 25 million starving people.